The Practice of Psychosocial Occupational Therapy

Linda Finlay

SECOND EDITION

Stanley Thornes (Publishers) Ltd

First published as *Occupational Therapy Practice in Psychiatry*
First edition published by Chapman & Hall in 1987
(ISBN 0-412-79910-3)

Second edition published 1997 by:
Stanley Thornes (Publishers) Ltd
Ellenborough House
Wellington Street
CHELTENHAM
GL50 1YW
United Kingdom

99 00 01 / 10 9 8 7 6 5 4 3 2

A catalogue record for this book is available from the British Library

ISBN 0-7487-3342-6

Typeset by Northern Phototypesetting Co Ltd., Bolton
Printed and bound in Great Britain by TJ International, Padstow, Cornwall

Contents

Case illustrations

Preface

I wrote the first edition of this textbook 10 years ago. Now, a decade on, it looks like a historical document(!) – the point that spurred me to undertake this major rewrite. As I compare the two editions, I find the changes extraordinary. The comparison gives a sharp sense of our professional history almost as it unfolds. Whilst there have been many continuities in our practice over the decade, the changes have been striking – changes which reflect major shifts in both the wider health care context and our professional education.

These changes which have had a profound impact on our practice can be summarised as follows. Firstly, the shifting health care context towards both the development of Trusts and more community practice has opened up different ways of working within treatment teams. Alongside changing health care policies we have had new imperatives to tighten up on our standards of practice, and we are now much more conscious of the need to measure and document outcomes and use standardised assessment measures. Then the expansion of degrees (and higher degrees) for professional training has coincided with a huge interest in research and an explosion in the use of occupational therapy theories and models. All of these changes have taken place in wider social context of changing demographics, new technologies and evolving cultural (even multi-cultural) practices.

I have tried to reflect these changes in this second edition. All the chapters have been largely re-written to accommodate new research and additional case illustrations. Plus, a completely new chapter on occupational therapy theory and models has been added.

The fact that this new edition is almost twice as long as the first demonstrates how much has been added. However, I hope I have also retained both the style and approach of the first edition. I still emphasise the need to be reflective practitioners who work systematically, but sensitively, through the stages of the occupational therapy process. I continue to stress the importance of being clear about our aims of practice and our options for achieving them using a sound theoretical foundation. This second edition builds on my previous message that we should be client-centred in our focus on occupational performance and our use of activity in treatment.

To this end, Chapter 1 takes an overview of our occupational therapy role in mental health, identifying core elements of our contribution to the treatment team.

Chapters 2 and 3 lay down our theoretical foundation exploring the use of occupational therapy models and different psychological approaches. Chapters 4, 5, 7 and 8 logically progress through the occupational therapy process of assessment, planning, implementation and evaluation of treatment. Each of these chapters is designed to offer specific guidelines of what the stage entails and how to carry it through. Chapter 6 extends the discussion on how to plan treatment and emphasises our special – even unique – focus on occupation and how to use activity therapeutically. Chapter 9 concludes by examining a range of more general discussions and debates surrounding our present and future practice.

I have tried to capture and reflect the diversity of our occupational therapy practice. To do this I offer a range of case examples which take place in various settings – hospital, community and specialist units, encompassing the use of both general and specialist techniques (e.g. craft work and ADL activities at one end of the spectrum to playtherapy and psychodrama at the other). Some of the case illustrations will fit the way you work – others will not be relevant. Hopefully there will be something for everyone to dip into according to interest.

Throughout the book I have emphasised the practical application of occupational therapy. To this end, many case studies and practical examples are used – indeed the whole of Chapter 7 is devoted to a series of case illustrations. In addition, the majority of chapters contain some 'theory into practice' boxes which explicitly highlight these 'how-to-do' aspects of the subject under discussion.

I have also sought to acknowledge and highlight those areas of our practice which are open to debate, e.g. whether or not we use particular theories or standardised assessment. It would be plainly wrong to attempt to offer some definitive statement of psychosocial occupational therapy, given both the variety of practice that exists and our philosophy of ensuring individualised treatments. Thus while I often give my personal view, I have also tried to allow for differing standpoints. The discussion questions at the end of each chapter may prove fruitful in encouraging further thought, discussion and debate.

Having outlined what this book is intended to do I would like also to mention its limits. Somewhat reluctantly I have restricted its scope to psychosocial practice primarily arising in the mental health field. I have not covered areas of physical handicap and learning disabilities, as these are areas in their own right which require full and separate treatment to do justice to the issues they raise. However, I see psychosocial occupational therapy has a role in both these other fields, and many of the principles and processes discussed throughout will have a general relevance to all areas of practice. Further, there are clear overlaps in all the areas – for instance when we work with elderly people, individuals with neurological disorders or developmentally delayed children. Some of the case studies offered reflect these overlaps, but I am conscious I have not done justice to the full spectrum of our practice.

In conclusion I would like to acknowledge a number of people who contributed to making this second edition. I wish to thank Ruth MacDonald and Sally Fowler Davis for their invaluable comments on my first draft; and Peter Gray, Janet

Gollege and Chris Mayers for their constructive advice. I also wish to express my thanks to Mel Wilder, without whose special and continuing support I would not have been able to write this edition. Finally, my gratitude needs to be extended to Neal Marriott, List Development Manager, and Serena Bureau, Editorial Assistant, Stanley Thornes who ably steered the final draft through to its completion, and Louise Watson, Senior Editor, for taking the manuscript on to publication. Needless to say, in the last analysis I alone remain responsible for any errors of content that may be found in the following pages.

Occupational therapy role in mental health | 1

Occupational therapists often find it hard to explain their role succinctly because of the huge diversity of practice. We can work in general or specialist units, in either hospitals or in the community. We treat people with all sorts of problems and needs, spanning individuals who have minor coping difficulties to those who are acutely ill or those with chronic, continuing disorders. In some units we employ groupwork activities and craft work, whilst in others we engage in one-to-one counselling. Our eclectic base offers us a choice of multiple theories, models of practice and assessment/treatment tools. Is there any common factor between occupational therapists who engage in such diverse practice? Are we able to articulate an occupational therapy role in mental health?

This chapter sets out to answer these questions. First, I review six core elements (aims and values) of occupational therapy. Then a second section develops this discussion to consider the role of occupational therapy within the multi-disciplinary team. It offers ideas about our unique contribution versus our shared values and how our division of labour can be negotiated. The third section briefly analyses the role of occupational therapy in different health care contexts. Here I try to convey something of the wide range of psychosocial practice. A final discussion section touches on some topical debates and confusions surrounding our role.

1.1 DEFINING OCCUPATIONAL THERAPY: CORE ELEMENTS

In common with the majority of occupational therapists I have some difficulty in defining our profession succinctly, in a way that captures the essence of what we do. First, our practice is diverse: we can be involved in so many different areas, working with individuals impaired psychologically, socially and physically. We seek to identify complex and varied problems of these individuals, and help them rebuild their lives in ways which are meaningful to them. This diversity of needs leads to a diversity of solutions and a variety of therapeutic roles. We also carry out such a variety of tasks from supplying a wheelchair, to baking a cake, to offering psychotherapy. Secondly, the value of our work is hard to quantify as often we deal with subjective and abstract processes such as the therapeutic relationship or the satisfaction gained through doing an activity.

All these features make it difficult to capture our practice, but it is still possible to identify some common aims and values. The exact nature of these core aims and values have been the subject of hot debate in our literature over the last 10 years, but I believe the following six elements reflect a consensus in the profession.

1. **Occupational performance.** Occupational therapists are centrally concerned with how individuals function in their work, leisure and domestic/personal self-care, i.e. their occupational performance. In our eyes we see a healthy person is one who is able to perform his or her daily occupations to a satisfying and effective level. A person's occupational performance may well be disrupted or impaired when he or she becomes ill or handicapped in some way. We work with these individuals who experience some difficulty in their daily life functioning.

2. **Importance of being active.** Occupational therapists believe that people are innately active beings. Through being active we learn about our selves, develop skills and maintain our physical/mental health. Reilly (1962, p. 2) captured this idea well in her statement, 'Man through the use of his hands as energised by mind and will, can influence the state of his own health'.

3. **Therapeutic use of activities.** Occupational therapy is premised on the idea that purposeful activity can be therapeutic and can be used to improve individuals' functioning. We apply activities in the treatment process valuing the activity's inherent properties, the experience of 'doing' and the end-product. We employ two main types of therapeutic activities: *activities of daily living* (ADL) (such as cooking) and specifically orientated *therapy activities* (such as groupwork). Treatment involves grading and adapting the activity and its inherent properties.

4. **Problem-solving process.** The occupational therapy process is primarily a problem-solving process (Hopkins and Tiffany, 1983). The first stage of the process is *assessment*, where we aim to identify an individual's problems of functioning. We then *plan treatment* by considering numerous options of what could be done to enhance a person's occupational performance. We consider the individual's skills, needs and lifestyle, and select the most promising problem-solving strategy that can be realistically applied, for *the implementation of treatment* stage. We then *evaluate* the treatment process, being alert to the need for further problem solving if necessary (see Figure 1.1). This process is a complex one where each stage blends into the next (e.g. from the first moment we enter into assessing individuals we simultaneously engage them in treatment).

5. **Holistic gaze.** Occupational therapists aim to view and treat individuals as complex, whole beings rather than homing in on isolated parts. We try to attend

to emotional, cognitive, social and physical aspects of the person. As Christiansen and Baum express it, 'Because of occupational therapy's focus on life performance, it is neither somatic, nor psychological, but concerned with the unity of body and mind in doing' (1991, p. 9). The fact that our professional training encompasses both physical and psychosocial aspects of health enables us to look widely at an individual's experience.

6. **Unique individuals.** Closely linked to our aim to see the 'whole' person, we value the uniqueness of each individual. Each person is seen to have his or her own skills, problems, needs, motives as well as a wider social and cultural heritage. The implications this carries for occupational therapy are that each person requires his or her own individualised treatment programme, one which cannot effectively be used for another. It also means that we resist (as far as possible) stereotyping our patients/clients (e.g. we avoid moral evaluations or categorising a person simply in terms of a diagnosis).

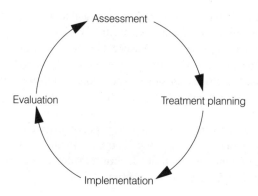

Figure 1.1 The occupational therapy process.

Taking the above core elements into account we can define occupational therapy as: **a holistic, problem-solving process which involves the therapeutic use of activities to enable individuals to perform their daily occupations to a satisfying and effective level.**

1.2 OCCUPATIONAL THERAPY ROLE WITHIN THE TEAM

Our occupational therapy role cannot be viewed in isolation. For one thing, the role we adopt is in part determined by the roles other team members adopt. So how do the key elements of occupational therapy operate given the multi-disciplinary team context? Do we have a unique contribution to make or are our values shared and acted upon by other team members?

Does occupational therapy have a unique contribution?

Creek (1996) offers a succinct and elegant summary of our contribution when she states, 'The uniqueness of the occupational therapy approach to psychosocial dysfunction lies in the philosophy of human beings having the ability to influence their own health through occupation' (p. 32). Basically, our central concern with *occupation and activity* provides us with a unique focus and role (i.e. the core elements 1–3 above). Here are two quotes from the literature reinforcing this point:

> The practice of occupational therapy involves 'the treatment of illness or disability through the analysis and use of the occupations which fill up a person's time and space and engage the individual in activity' (Reed and Sanderson, 1983).

> 'Occupational therapy is the use of purposeful activity and interventions to promote health and achieve functional outcomes' (American Occupational Therapy Association, 1994).

Whilst nurses and other professionals may attend to activities of daily living (e.g. during the nursing process) and use activities in treatment (e.g. when physiotherapists offer group exercises), these aspects do not constitute their primary focus. We privilege occupation and activity – they do not. In a similar way, occupational therapists might encroach on other professionals' territory: we might work on managing a person's mental state (really the central domain of doctors and nurses using a medical model) or we could choose to utilise a systematic desensitisation programme (normally the province of the psychologist) or offer psychotherapy (in pure terms the area for those specifically trained in this). All of these interventions could be part of a therapeutic tool bag, but they do not constitute the main thrust of an occupational therapist's contribution.

Shared values within the team

I have sometimes heard it argued that occupational therapy is unique in that we offer a holistic, problem-solving process which focuses on treating individuals (i.e. encompassing core elements 4–6 above). I disagree. These values do not make us unique and I would suggest that to say so makes us sound a touch arrogant. To a greater or lesser extent all team members share these values. Doctors (and many nurses) experience a 'dual' training and are therefore at least as 'holistic' as occupational therapists. Also, all team members engage in a problem-solving process – in fact the very term occupational therapy process (assessment, treatment planning, etc.) was taken from 'The Nursing Process'.

Team members not only share similar values about problem solving, it seems we also tend to employ similar forms of clinical reasoning that is both technical/rational reasoning and 'reflection in action' (Schon, 1983). In other words, we all engage in a combination of logic and intuitive, instinctive experience. However, the precise form this thinking takes is likely to be profession specific.

For example, on observing a patient who has a violent outburst, a doctor might review what sedating medication would be suitable; a nurse might explore how best to contain and manage the behaviour; an occupational therapist might wonder what activity seemed to precipitate the outburst or what has a calming effect. Of course, in reality it is not quite as simple and clear cut as this as all the professionals involved would analyse the situation at different levels. I am merely suggesting certain profession specific themes are likely to predominate.

Given the above points I think it is more accurate to say that the aims of the *multi-disciplinary* team are to engage in a holistic, problem-solving process – one individual professional cannot hope to look at all aspects of a person. It is only as a team that we can really come close to achieving 'holistic' treatment, allowing different members to focus on different aspects of need in different ways.

Team working

In order to achieve the holistic practice described above, one decision a team needs to make is to establish the different roles of the professionals involved. Often teams opt for a division of labour between members whereby each professional focuses on a different aspect of the patient's/client's treatment. For instance, it is common to see a pattern where nurses take on the acute care and behavioural management of a newly admitted patient, whilst the occupational therapist focuses on looking at longer term issues related to discharge. Alternatively, the team may select a model of working where roles are blurred and the professionals involved act as generic or 'key' workers (a pattern most frequently seen in Community Mental Health teams).

More commonly, teams operate a combination of these two positions, where a certain amount of role blurring is accepted but key workers are chosen to fit the professional's particular skills and interests. For instance the occupational therapist might specialise in patients/clients with particular occupational performance difficulties, whilst the nurses take on cases where long-term medication management is the problematic issue.

The fact that roles often need to be negotiated within a team means that an element of competition can arise between members. One professional group may feel they are not being valued as highly as another. Sometimes professionals can become territorial and defensive about their role. How many times do we hear irritation being expressed that another professional has taken over what should have been 'our job'?!

There are no easy solutions to combat problems of team working as staff dynamics and internal politics can be powerful factors. However, I feel we are in a stronger position if we remember, and act upon, three things:

1. We should maintain our core values and skills (i.e. our focus on occupational performance.

2. When other team members focus on or use 'activity' we should see this as a compliment and not a threat.
3. Ultimately we need to keep focused on the central question: Is the patient/client getting 'a good deal' from the way the team is functioning (whatever the division of labour)?

1.3 ROLE OF OCCUPATIONAL THERAPY IN DIFFERENT HEALTH CARE CONTEXTS

Not only does our occupational therapy role depend on the team approach, it varies according to the needs of the particular patient/client group involved and the treatment context. I find it useful to distinguish between the role of occupational therapy in hospitals versus the role in the community; and in terms of various specialist roles. Each of these three areas will be briefly described in turn. See Table 1.1.

Before doing this, let me emphasise the point that my distinction between hospital, community and specialist roles is artificial, and that often the 'real world' is not so clear cut. The areas overlap and link (e.g. many individuals live in the community but attend a day hospital or we might see a relatively healthy individual in a primary care context who is later admitted to hospital, acutely ill). Also, whilst I separate out specialist roles, these always take place in either hospital or community settings and are not usually divorced from general practice.

Table 1.1 Comparing hospital and community occupational therapy roles

Hospital roles	Community roles
Acute admission units	Primary care
contain behaviour	health education
teach coping strategies	support
assessment	teach coping strategies
Middle/long-stay units	Continuing care
maintenance	support of individuals and carers
develop functional skills	mobilise community resources
rehabilitation	monitor mental state and progress

Hospital roles

Acute admission

People who are admitted to hospital are usually severely ill/disturbed. They are often a danger to themselves (e.g. they might be a suicide risk) or others (e.g. they might be violent or unpredictable). Their ability to cope with everyday life is usually severely impaired – though perhaps only temporarily – by extreme feelings (such as anxiety) or disturbed cognitive-perceptual processes (such as delusions). Patients are often discharged home or transferred within a month. This time-scale significantly affects our hospital role as therapy needs to be applied promptly.

Occupational therapists are limited in what they can do when a patient is acutely ill. The actual medical/psychiatric condition and symptomatology (e.g. delusions and hallucinations) is often best treated by medication. Our role is usually limited to offering activities which help *contain* the person's behaviour (such as using concrete, relaxing activities to help the person focus on the here and now). We also have an *assessment function* to observe the person whilst he or she is engaged in activity. Often such assessment can assist with differential diagnosis decisions.

Our biggest role with acute admission patients is when they are getting better and need to be prepared to return to their home environment. After carefully assessing their problems and situation we might offer a range of treatments geared to *giving support and offering coping strategies*. The most commonly used treatments which can take place on the ward or in a department are:

- Anxiety management training to learn practical coping skills.
- Practical or craft activities to promote productive behaviour, social contact and self-esteem.
- Dramatherapy or other groupwork to gain support and learn from others.

As soon as patients 'feel better' they are discharged – and sometimes earlier than that. Assessing the optimum time for discharge (given pressures of needing spare beds) is a crucial decision the team needs to make. We have an important function to ensure patients are *safe to return home* and adequately prepared to cope with their expected environment. Perhaps our most useful function in the acute setting is to *offer on-going out-patient support* bridging the gap between hospital and community.

Middle/long stay

People in this category include both those who receive treatment over several months and those who have stayed in (or moved in and out of) the hospital system for years as part of a 'revolving door' system. These patients/clients typically suffer a continuing handicap (such as having a psychotic, affective or organic disorder with associated functional problems) and characteristically display additional problems of institutionalisation (passivity, dependence and apathy). Usually all areas of their occupational performance (work, domestic, leisure and self-care) are impaired. These problems are further exacerbated by the appalling, hostile social environments, including unemployment, poverty, lack of social support, within which individuals in this group are forced to live.

The main occupational therapy aim with this group is to maintain or develop *independence* and *functional skills*. A range of treatment activities can be utilised involving all areas of:

- Personal – self-presentation and self-care.
- Domestic/work – home management and other productive work tasks.
- Social – social skills training and hobby interests.

The focus throughout is on *rehabilitation and resettlement* where possible (e.g. to a group home or day centre). It is important to be realistic about the long-term aims with this group of patients. Aiming to resettle someone into full-time employment is not only unrealistic, but likely to be too pressured and ultimately destructive to the individual. Sheltered work or craft activities available in a long-term day centre placement would be ideal to offer a daily structure and work role. Occupational therapists, alongside other team members, may also work with the patients'/clients' family or carers offering both *support and advice*.

Community roles

The implementation of Griffiths' report, *Community Care: An Agenda for Action*, has meant a gradual (and continuing) shift of resources away from the National Health Service. The report distinguishes between medical and social care, and encourages a shift in emphasis from illness to health models. Increasingly, it is being recognised that people with continuing mental health problems can fall between hospital and community services. The concept of 'spectrum of care' is beginning to replace 'community care'.

'Normality' is a concept which is emphasised in social care models. One theory which focuses on such ideas is 'normalisation theory' (also called Social Role Valorization by Wolfensberger, 1983). Its central concern is with the rights of mentally disabled people to live a full life in the community. The theory suggests that much disability is socially created (by poor services and negative public images) and that a person's competency will be enhanced by engaging in 'normal' activities. Thus, going with a patient to the local swimming baths is seen as more appropriate than using hospital gym facilities.

With the large mental hospitals closing (involving the loss of thousands of psychiatric in-patient beds), more and more people are being treated in their own homes or day care settings. Community Mental Health Teams (CMHTs) have mushroomed in each district/region. The radical changes in care which have occurred in the last decade, has meant the field is still new and community treatment teams are still exploring their roles and parameters. Each CMHT seems to work differently and respond to different local needs. Some teams emphasise skill mix and operate a division of labour according to professional roles; other teams recommend role blurring and a 'case manager' approach. Some teams focus on primary mental health care where treatment largely involves one-to-one supportive counselling to prevent mental illness and takes place in the client's home. Other community teams offer continuing care and rehabilitation and work often takes place in special day care/drop-in centres. Here is how two different Community Occupational Therapists describe their roles.

Primary care

I work with people who have mental health problems as opposed to being mentally ill. They tend to be in crisis and need to 'off-load' or simply need some extra support to cope … We all try to avoid diagnostic labels and see the client as an individual within their home environment. Having said that I group my clients into: (a) people with anxiety related problems, (b) people with relationship problems (marriage, children, etc.) and (c) people with particular emotional problems related to trauma for instance bereavement or sexual abuse. My main roles are that of key worker and counsellor. As a key worker I manage their case and follow through relevant referrals, etc. As a counsellor I usually see people individually at home or in the unit, for an hour long weekly or fortnightly session. I also run a weekly anxiety management group with a CPN. Some people I only see a few times; others I follow-up for many months depending on what we both feel might be beneficial.

I suppose that my occupational therapy training gives me a particular slant when working with a client, but I see myself more as a case worker. Having said that the team uses our particular strengths – mine is running groups which goes back to my occupational therapy training. The CPNs tend to work more with people who need injections or their medication monitored and we all do counselling.

Continuing care

I see my role in terms of being a member of a Community Rehabilitation Team. Usually our clients have a history of mental illness and it is our job to give support and maintain them for as long as possible in the community. As a community therapist I have a role to monitor clients' mental health (e.g. to ensure they are taking their medication and are generally coping). For this we do regular (fairly brief) home visit checks. We also offer a drop-in service at our centre for people to get immediate help if they feel they are having problems.

My role as an occupational therapist specifically is to look at a person's activities of daily living in the work, social and domestic areas. Often the key factor which separates clients who cope and those who return to hospital is whether or not they are involved in meaningful occupations. Having something to do gives them a structure to their day and helps them feel effective and worthwhile. I co-ordinate any community services that might be needed like it might be setting up day centre attendance or arranging a support group for the carers. Twice weekly I'm involved in running different occupational therapy groups at the local day hospital.

Specialist roles

A number of occupational therapists work in specialist units (e.g. in child and family psychiatry or forensic psychiatry). It is not possible to reflect the full range of specialist practice; however, the following descriptions offer a flavour of our different roles. See Table 1.2.

Table 1.2 Specialist occupational therapy roles

Working with children	playtherapy stimulate developmental skills and functioning
Working with elderly people	assess safe ADL functioning offer stimulating cognitive and social activities
Working with people with learning disabilities	sensori-motor activities to stimulate development and skills facilitate occupational performance act as the client's advocate habilitation and resettlement
Working in forensic psychiatry	provide containing activities to manage violent or disturbed acute behaviour community resettlement and reintegration
Working in substance abuse units	offer therapeutic activities to explore managing the substance abuse problem time and leisure management

Working with children

Play, in all its forms, is arguably the most significant occupation for children. For this reason, most occupational therapists working with children act as playtherapists. The therapist might utilise a psychodynamic or humanistic framework and offer *playtherapy* sessions (e.g. free play opportunities) to encourage the child to express and explore his or her feelings. Alternatively, the therapist might be more concerned with the child's *developmental functioning* and would use play to develop the child's cognitive, motor and social skills.

Perhaps the biggest difference between working with children and adults is that when treating a child, greater emphasis is placed on the family (who both affects and is affected by the child). Many occupational therapists who work in child and family psychiatry units will get involved in treating the family at some level. The therapist might aim to teach the parents *basic parenting skills* or how to play with the child. The therapist might also participate in *family therapy* sessions, often in conjunction with other team members.

Working with people who are elderly

Elderly people comprise a significant portion of the work of many occupational therapists both in general practice (e.g. where someone has become depressed) or in our work within specialist units. Arguably, our professional training equips us with skills which are especially relevant for treating elderly people as they often experience multiple problems (due in part to the effects of ageing) where it is difficult to separate emotional, cognitive, social and physical dimensions.

When occupational therapists work in specialist units for elderly people, the units commonly fall into two basic categories: short-term assessment units and long-stay (hospital or day) units.

People might be referred to the assessment-type unit for a short admission – usually in order to identify a diagnosis and/or to assess the person's level of safety. Occupational therapists play a crucial role in determining if/when a person is *'safe' to return home*. This typically involves assessing their cooking ability and independence in self-care. We would also attempt to investigate the person's wider occupational performance (e.g. looking at the individual's use of time and whether or not they engage in meaningful, satisfying *leisure* pursuits).

Occupational therapists who work in the longer stay units usually focus on the individual's cognitive and social functioning (e.g. offering **reality orientation** and **reminiscence therapy**). Along with other members of the team we would be concerned to provide *activities* and stimulation designed to maintain the individual's functioning and independence, as well as providing enjoyment and opportunities for social interaction.

Working with people who have learning disabilities

Arguably learning disabilities is a field in itself and not a 'specialism'; however, when looking at the broad sweep of psychosocial occupational therapy it can be regarded as a specialist area.

People with learning disabilities have a range of needs depending on their level of disability and functioning. Whilst we seek to avoid unduly categorising people, it is possible to distinguish between those individuals who are profoundly and multiply handicapped and may need life-long institutional care, and those with special needs (e.g. education) who can live relatively independent, if sheltered, lives in the community given some support.

The occupational therapists role with individuals who are profoundly and/or multiply handicapped is varied. The therapist might utilise a range of sensorimotor *activities* designed to stimulate and develop skills. Music and other activities involving light, movement, noise and touch are commonly used to stimulate sensory awareness. In addition, the occupational therapist may be involved in supplying a range of *adaptive equipment* towards treating any physical disabilities and increasing functional ability (e.g. to assist an individual to sit or eat independently). As a member of the team the therapist may also be involved in implementing a range of programmes to manage 'problem' behaviour and develop skills.

The occupational therapist's role with more independent individuals with learning disabilities is equally varied. Essentially the occupational therapist acts in the capacities of teacher, facilitator and advocate. As a *teacher/facilitator*, the therapist aims to develop the individual's skills – cognitive, social and practical (in terms of daily functioning). As the client's *advocate*, the therapist will endeavour to protect the individual's interests and encourage him or her to make personal choices. Both roles may require the occupational therapist to work with carers (e.g. to reduce any tendency to be over-protective) and the local community (e.g. dealing with hostile social responses).

Therapists will often be involved in the long term (habilitation rather than rehabilitation), e.g. *resettling* the client to live independently or in a sheltered housing scheme. In such circumstances the person's wider occupational performance will need attention – both to develop skills and facilitate opportunities for work and leisure.

Forensic psychiatry

The forensic occupational therapist has special skills and experience in dealing with violent, disturbed behaviour. The role of occupational therapy in forensic psychiatry is as diverse as in general psychiatry. Occupational therapists who specialise in this area may work in hospitals (secure areas), in the community or in specialist secure units (liaising with the prison service).

Sometimes the patients/clients are acutely ill (e.g. actively hallucinating). In these situations the therapist will be largely involved in supplying *containing activities* and could offer some social skills training (e.g. with a focus on managing anger). Forensic therapists are also involved in long-term rehabilitation where treatment focuses on developing the person's skills and *community resettlement/reintegration*.

Substance abuse units

The occupational therapist who specialises in treating people who abuse drugs or alcohol works closely with the other team members in following the unit's treatment philosophy (e.g. controlled drinking programmes versus total abstinence). The team will endeavour to engage and keep the patient/client in treatment (which involves encouraging his or her motivation to change). In addition, the occupational therapist might offer specific *therapeutic activities* such as projective art (paint what alcohol means) or social skills training (e.g. saying 'no' to a drink). Otherwise the occupational therapist will focus on the person's longer term occupational performance. In particular attention is usually paid to *managing time/leisure* when trying to replace the alcohol consumption or drug use.

1.4 DEBATES AND REFLECTIONS ABOUT THE OCCUPATIONAL THERAPY ROLE

So far I have presented the occupational therapy role as being relatively clear-cut and unproblematic. The reality of our 'search' for a unifying professional identity and to be valued within the team offers a somewhat different picture. No discussion about the occupational therapy role can be complete without some acknowledgement that there are debates about the purpose and form our role should take. Confusions about this can be found both within our profession and amongst others outside (i.e. our patients/clients and other team members).

Debates within occupational therapy

Within occupational therapy, we do not yet have (and maybe never will) a consensus about our priorities. Should we favour working in hospitals or the community? Should we concentrate on working with acutely ill or more chronically impaired people (to say nothing about working with the 'worried well'!). Should we utilise groupwork and activities in treatment or should we emphasise a one-to-one counselling role? Should we focus on 'occupation' or on the teaching and learning of 'skills'. Should we utilise a plurality of theories and models or keep focused on one?

None of these questions have easy answers and therapists will vary in their opinions. In my view we should focus our attention on areas where we can be most effective and make the most impact. This will differ in different units/contexts. By- and-large I favour maintaining our focus on our aims of assisting occupational performance. This would usually imply some level of community involvement. It also suggests we should be cautious about embracing 'non-occupational therapy' interventions, such as becoming involved with medication and (pure) counselling, without further training. Whatever role is undertaken I believe that all therapists need to be clear and confident about their role. Then, rather than being self-absorbed and feeling uncertain or defensive about their contribution, they will be able to give their full attention to the needs of their patients/clients. In much the same way our choice of theoretical base and aims of treatment should be established with patients/clients in mind.

Confusions about occupational therapy

Time and again we are confronted by the fact that patients/clients and other professionals do not sufficiently understand what occupational therapy is all about. Whilst a number of studies (e.g. Stockwell et al., 1987) have shown that patients/clients value occupational therapy, it appears they also have a number of misconceptions. Harries and Caan (1994) demonstrated how patients seem to see occupational therapy as providing entertainment, keeping them busy or even giving the ward staff a break(!). Polimeni-Walker, Wilson and Jewens (1992) studying practice in the US found patients similarly valued the diversional element of occupational therapy.

My reaction to findings like these is three-fold. First, I am pleased patients/clients seem to value our services. Then, I wonder what kind of experience of occupational therapy they have had. Was the occupational therapist clear about what was being offered? Did the therapist negotiate treatment aims and objectives with the individual? I also wonder if patients/clients have indeed appreciated a deeper significance and value of occupational therapy, but find it hard to articulate, so settle for easy definitions like being occupied.

A number of other studies demonstrate team members vary in their understanding of the occupational therapy role. One study by Jenkins and Brotherton (1995) demonstrates marked variations in views about occupational therapy amongst both occupational therapy staff and other team members. Smith (1986) found doctors had a limited understanding of occupational therapy. Harries and Caan (1994) showed how ward staff on a psychiatric unit were not adverse to seeing occupational therapy in terms of entertainment. More positively, Kaur, Slager and Orrell (1996) surveyed attitudes to occupational therapy of 89 mental health staff in a psychiatric unit. Whilst many staff were well able to recognise key occupational therapy functions, they were not confident about their knowledge and did not apply it in their practice (e.g. in referral patterns).

Clearly we have an ongoing 'battle' on our hands to promote what we do and to resist being perceived as simply 'entertainment' or 'diversion'. I feel it is down to us as a professional group to educate others and clarify what we do. We have to take some responsibility when others have negative images of our role. Perhaps these images are based on a reality? In the last analysis I think it is impressive that so many professionals have an idea of what occupational therapists do, given the enormous changes that have taken place in our role and functions in the last 30 years. The fact that they value our contribution is even more rewarding!

Discussion questions

1. Analyse the core elements of occupational therapy.
2. Do occupational therapists have a unique contribution to make?
3. To what extent is occupational therapy holistic in practice?
4. 'Role blurring between the occupational therapist and other team members creates only problems and confusions'. Discuss.
5. Discuss the view that 'there is little point in occupational therapists treating people who are acutely ill'.
6. The Louis Blom-Cooper report (1989) recommended that 80% of occupational therapists who work in hospitals should be re-deployed in the community sector. Do you agree that this is an effective move forward for both occupational therapists and their clients?

Occupational therapy theory and models

2

When you are asked 'how would you treat a particular client?', do you respond that it depends on how you analyse his or her problem – that somehow a 'right' analysis will lead to a 'right' way to treat the person? Unfortunately, things are not so straightforward. Our treatments depend on many factors: the health care context, team policy, practical constraints and, arguably most significantly, which theoretical perspective is adopted. That theoretical perspective (in the form of theory or model) gives us our 'spectacles' through which we view our patients/clients, their needs and problems, and the occupational therapy process. It helps us know what to look for and what to treat. It also gives us an understanding of how and why we carry our certain treatments.

Both this chapter and the next are designed to persuade therapists who may be reluctant to explore 'theory' that some theoretical rational is necessary – both for our profession and for effective practice. I will attempt to do this, in this chapter, by first drawing our theoretical context in broad brush strokes, then describing four of our most widely used models. The next section takes five case illustrations and demonstrates how the models are applied in practice. The final section outlines a few key ideas from other relevant occupational therapy theories. It is of course impossible to do justice to any of these theories and models in just one chapter, so I strongly recommend you return to the original source materials to gain a deeper understanding. Chapter 3 will continue exploring our use of theory by analysing how psychological approaches are applied.

2.1 THE THEORETICAL CONTEXT

Why have theory?

Theory, models and frames of reference are our 'mental filing cabinets' (Yerxa, 1987) which help us organise our knowledge. More than this, they allow us to communicate knowledge and understanding to others. Theory is often used unconsciously or implicitly, but the value of applying some theoretical base self-consciously, however, can be seen at a number of levels.

1. *A guide to practice.* When we are faced with the daunting task of treating another human being with all his or her complexities, our theoretical framework gives us a place to start and a way of moving forward. Further, we need some theory base to encourage coherent and systematic treatment. Without it we risk 'synthesising a plan for therapy that contains contradictory assumptions and modes of practice' (Briggs *et al.*, 1979, p. 2). An example here is the use of reward star charts (behavioural strategy) with a child, whilst using non-directive playtherapy (humanistic strategy) simultaneously.

2. *A guide to alternative practice.* Different theories often define the problems differently and suggest alternative treatment strategies. Being aware of other theories/perspectives helps us to reflect on, critique and evaluate our work.

3. *A tool to encourage team co-operation.* If we are ignorant of the theoretical biases within the team our opportunities to blend treatment co-operatively, and to communicate effectively, are lessened. It follows both that any divisions between the team members may arise because they are subscribing to different theoretical frameworks and that if we want to challenge existing practice we need to understand others' positions.

4. *A way forward for the profession.* A theoretical base provides both a rationale and method for documenting and researching our practice. This is vital, given increasing demands for accountability. 'A well-developed theoretical structure allows the therapist to meet questions from administrators, other professionals, families, clients and perhaps most importantly, questions that may arise from oneself as a therapist' (Fidler and Fidler, 1983, p. 292). Can we even call ourselves professional if we do not have a coherent, logical, theoretical framework within which to work?

Defining terms and concepts

Currently there is much confusion and corresponding debate surrounding definitions of terms such as models, theories, approaches, frames of reference. Pick up any book concerned with occupational therapy theory and the author seems to present another view! We have Reed (1984) and Kielhofner (1992) who both focus on 'models', but disagree as to what they are. For instance, Reed attempts to encompass all our theory under the banner of models, whereas Kielhofner prefers to link them more specifically with occupational therapy practice. Kielhofner's conceptual practice model parallels what Mosey (1981) describes as a frame of reference (though she is largely referring to theories borrowed from other disciplines and applied to occupational therapy). In Australia, Kortman (1994) distinguishes between professional, delineation and applications models. In the UK, Creek (1996), Hagedorn (1995, 1996) and Mayers (1990), amongst others, have entered into the fray with their own definitions. At the risk of confusing you further, I would like to offer you my simplified schema of how some of these concepts, theories and models fit together. For deeper, more sophisticated explorations I would strongly recommend you return to the references above.

In order to avoid potential confusion surrounding terms, let me start by laying out my definitions of the main words.

Theory	A system of assumptions and principles devised to analyse, predict or explain behaviour or experience (or other phenomena).
Model	A simplified representation of a phenomenon that can account for certain data/relationships (e.g. we can have a model of human development or a model of occupational therapy practice).
Frame of reference	Our general orientation, a collection of ideas or theories which provide a foundation for practice.
Approach	The method or way of putting a chosen theory into practice.
Philosophy	Our fundamental beliefs, guiding precepts and values.
Paradigm	Broad philosophical movements (e.g. positivist, mechanistic paradigm versus naturalistic, holistic paradigm) – it is the profession's 'world view' (Creek and Feaver, 1993).

Having defined these terms, let me emphasise one point. Ultimately it is the content of these concepts/theories which are important. Rather than getting side-tracked into semantics and trying to define the terms, I would recommend that you recognise they are 'contested concepts' and move on. Only engage in the definitions debate once you have a reasonable understanding about what is being expressed by the different ideas and theories. Perhaps Kortman had the right idea when he declared, 'a model is a frame of reference is a paradigm is an approach'! Rather than getting caught up with meanings we should simply recognise their are different types of models: abstract to practical; broad to specific (Kortman, 1994).

Theoretical framework

Theory, model, frame of reference, approach, philosophy and paradigm – all interact in practice. When amalgamated they can be called our *theoretical framework* (see Figure 2.1).

Philosophy

We start with our fundamental professional beliefs and values, i.e. our philosophy. There are two essential strands to our philosophy. One, our philosophical base is essentially humanistic and client-centred (ideas which arise out of the naturalistic, holistic paradigm which rejects the reductionist and positivist tendencies of any mechanistic view of humans). We strive to view individuals holistically, seeing

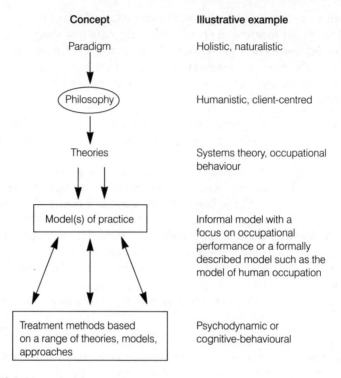

Figure 2.1 Theoretical framework.

them as active, autonomous, unique beings. Each individual has their own value and potential. Two, we also believe in the intrinsic value of activity and occupation. We believe that the drive to act is a basic human need. Moreover, we believe that an individual's health can be influenced by engaging in activity, so we exploit this in therapy. (See the six core elements of the occupational therapy role in Chapter 1.)

Models of practice

Our philosophy then 'feeds' our model(s) of practice – be they occupational therapy models or ones culled from other disciplines (e.g. when we use psychological approaches). These models act as our 'conceptual lenses' (Kielhofner, 1992) through which we can understand a person's function/dysfunction. They also can suggest a structure for clinical reasoning and how we might view the therapy process.

Our practice is always underpinned by models, though often we are unaware of them! For instance we routinely draw on broad sweep models such as a 'social model' (versus medical models) or a 'rehabilitation model' (which Ekdawi and Conning, 1994, divide into disability model, needs model and skills model).

Mental health teams routinely subscribe to psychodynamic and cognitive-behavioural models.

In terms of profession specific models, much debate (Kielhofner, 1992; Creek and Feaver, 1993; Hagedorn, 1996) has been taken up over the last decade defining and identifying our occupational therapy practice models. Many occupational therapists say they operate with implicit or even 'personal models' (Kortman, 1994). In terms of explicitly articulated models, four of the most widely and currently applied models in the UK are: the Model of Human Occupation (Kielhofner, 1985, 1995) the Canadian Occupational Performance Model (Canadian Association of Occupational Therapists, 1991), Reed's (1984) Adaptation through Occupation Model and Mosey's Adaptive Skills Model.

Treatment methods and approaches

Once we have established our particular focus (using a model as our spectacles), we then implement treatment. Here we can draw on a whole range of other theories, models, approaches. For example, we can apply a psychodynamic approach or implement a specific cognitive-behavioural treatment method. We can even bring in other practice models (e.g. Egan's, 1986, counselling model of 'the skilled helper'). So, the treatment methods we use can be based on other theories, but we draw on them as *therapeutic tools*. This use of theory will be explored in Chapter 3.

THEORY INTO PRACTICE

Case example: **The use of different theoretical frameworks**

Phil is a 42-year-old man who was made redundant from his job in the fishing industry 2 years ago and he has since been unemployed. His brother died of a drug overdose last year. Phil has had several bouts of depression in the past couple of years – and on the last occasion he was suicidal and needed to be hospitalised. Phil also has an alcohol problem which results in periodic drinking binges which last several days. During these times he becomes both morose and unpredictably aggressive. In addition to these problems he has become overweight which worsens his already negative self-image. He used to enjoy physical activity and sports, but now lacks the drive to be active. Phil lives in a small bedsit with his girlfriend and a one-year-old daughter who he adores (and whom he says is his main reason for living). His parents are supportive though they live a distance away and cannot offer much help financially.

Using the Model of Human Occupation

If we used the Model of Human Occupation as our spectacles through which to view Phil, his problems would be understood in terms of loss of work role/work habits which have resulted in volitional problems (low sense of personal causation and lack of valued activities/hobby interests). He is in a vicious cycle as he is not getting any positive feedback (both internally and externally related to the environment) on his occupational performance. Treatment might be directed towards encouraging Phil to engage more in valued occupations. One-to-one counselling or groupwork would be appropriate methods to use for him to explore and begin to act positively on his role needs and occupational interests.

Using a psychodynamic approach
If we took a psychodynamic approach, we would view Phil's priority problems in terms of his feelings, his unconscious needs and his relationships. We could focus on his multiple 'bereavements' and recognise all the major life stresses he has had to cope with recently from a lost job and death, to the birth of a new baby. We might also put the spotlight on his unconscious needs and his 'anger'. His relationships with his girlfriend, daughter and parents would be of particular relevance. The treatment of choice would be psychotherapy or perhaps some creative therapy activities (e.g. projective art).

Using a cognitive-behavioural approach
A therapist using a cognitive-behavioural approach would focus on how Phil seemed locked in a pattern of negative thinking which resulted in spiralling destructive behaviours – this could be explored in one-to-one counselling. Alternatively, Phil might benefit from groupwork (e.g. joining an assertiveness training group where he could learn to handle frustration positively). A behavioural contract could also be drawn up for him to abstain from drinking during his treatment.

All the approaches and treatments described above offer a positive way forward for Phil's treatment. Which one is the best or most appropriate approach for occupational therapy is a matter for debate and one we shall engage in later. The point to appreciate now is that none of the treatments described offer a comprehensive solution to all Phil's problems, i.e. they only deal with their particular focus. It is often the case that if one or two problems are resolved, the others will unravel in their own way. Thus, if Phil can feel positive about one thing, or succeed in one area of his life, he may well be able to marshall his resources to cope with his other problems.

A final point to bear in mind about having such a theoretical framework as I have described is that it is not static and different occupational therapists employ different versions at different times. Whilst I would say the majority of occupational therapists would subscribe to the philosophy outlined above, everything else is open for negotiation. Some therapists will use a range of occupational therapy models and treatment approaches; others prefer to work within one consistent theoretical framework, for instance taking a psychodynamic approach alongside other team members. Mostly therapists take an eclectic, pragmatic line on theory. They tend to go along with what is known as a post-modern trend to reject particular universal or grand theory and instead draw upon and integrate different theories. No wonder our theoretical base is complicated!

2.2 FOUR OCCUPATIONAL THERAPY MODELS

This section will analyse the key ideas of four of the most widely practised (and researched) 'models' of occupational therapy, i.e. the Model of Human Occupation (Kielhofner, 1985, 1995), the Occupational Performance Model (Canadian Association of Occupational Therapists, 1991), Adaptation through Occupation Model (Reed, 1984) and the Adaptive Skills Model (Mosey, 1970, 1986). All of these models themselves arise out of established theory (e.g. from the field of psychology including developmental and learning theories).

Side-stepping any debate about whether or not the four 'models' are in fact models (!), I have selected these on pragmatic grounds. First, they seem to be the major (occupational therapy) models therapists in the UK identify as being relevant. Secondly, they are all models which capture the essence of occupational therapy and reflect our practice concerns. Not surprisingly, they are, in some ways, remarkably similar. Finally, I have used each of these models in my clinical practice, so I am able to comment on both the theory and their practical applications.

I have tried to remain impartial in my judgements about which model is the 'best'. All the models have strengths and limitations. In principle, I believe it is a healthy sign that our profession can draw on several models, i.e. that we can select which appears to be most appropriate at any one time. Extra space has been given to examining the model of human occupation due to its greater complexity and extensive research base.

Before moving on to look at the models I would like to make one personal comment. I am hesitant that the fact of having chosen these four models in some ways puts them in 'tablets of stone'. This is not my intention. I envisage that all models will come and go. These are sure to be revised and replaced by other newer and (hopefully) better models. These four simply reflect our current professional development and practice. I sincerely hope that the next decade will bring more models to the fore – ideally with more research relevant to practice in the UK. As Creek puts it, 'Occupational therapy is a dynamic profession in a rapidly changing world; therefore it does not have a fixed, universally agreed model' (1996, p. 43). I would go further and say that if we are to remain a dynamic profession, our models must evolve and change, and what is more, we must be ready to change with them.

The Model of Human Occupation

Key concepts

The Model of Human Occupation (Kielhofner, 1995) can be summarised in terms of seven key concepts.

1. **Occupational behaviour.** Occupational behaviour is the focus of the model of

human occupation. Based on Reilly's occupational behaviour theory (see p. 40 in this chapter), the model stresses the central importance of activity and action. The model sees action, in the form of occupational behaviour, as fundamental to the growth and development of the system (i.e. the person). The need to be active is seen as programmed into human beings, arising spontaneously, i.e. by their nature people are disposed to act.

2. **Systems theory.** The model draws on many theories, in particular it draws on systems theory. The model conceptualises a human as being an open system (consisting of sub-systems) which operates within wider systems. Occupational behaviour is seen to result from a dynamic process where internal biological and psychological factors interact with the physical and socio-cultural world. A person is viewed as both influencing and being influenced by his or her environment.

3. **Interacting sub-systems.** Kielhofner conceptualises the human as being made of three interacting sub-systems: volition, habituation and performance. The key issue is how these sub-systems are seen to contribute to our occupational behaviour. The volition sub-system is seen as *choosing* the occupational behaviour – it gives us our energy, motivation, interest to engage in action. The habituation sub-system *organises* the behaviour into routines and patterns – it keeps us doing our occupational behaviour. The mind–brain–body performance sub-system gives us the skills to be able to *perform*, to carry out our occupational behaviour.

4. **The volition sub-system.** The volition sub-system encompasses both a kind of emotional disposition to act and self-knowledge (what we think of ourselves and our goals) which will influence how we anticipate, interpret and choose our occupations. This way of thinking/feeling includes three areas: (a) images about our own effectiveness (personal causation), (b) convictions about what is important and a sense of rights/obligations (values), and (c) an attraction towards and preference for certain occupations (interests). To illustrate how the volition sub-system affects occupational behaviour in practice consider: the person who 'feels a failure' and so avoids doing something as they fear further failure; or, as another example, a person may not want to do something, but does it because he or she feels it is important and should be done. One way people come to understand themselves is through telling stories – termed volitional narrative (see case illustration 2.2 on p. 34). These 'stories' arise in a cultural context and can influence behaviour.

5. **The habituation sub-system.** The habituation sub-system comprises of: (a) habits and habit map, and (b) internalised roles and scripts. Habits refer to the behavioural patterns and internalised images of how behaviour should be organised and operates mainly at a preconscious level. Roles involve an awareness of particular social identities related to social positions and how one is expected to behave. An example of the habituation sub-system in action is the way we behave when we go to work in the morning. We may not want to go but we go, because we have a role to fulfil (i.e. we know it is expected) and that

is our routine. A long holiday or sickness can interrupt our habitual pattern which means we need to work on developing new routines.

6. **Mind–brain–body performance sub-system.** The performance sub-system is conceptualised as the organiser of our capacity to perform and is made up of musculoskeletal, neurological, cardiopulmonary and symbolic (relevant for language, cognition and unconscious processing) elements. Whilst we cannot observe the system directly (e.g. our information processing capacity), we can make inferences about the state of the constituent's parts. An example of this is the person with some cognitive impairment who is unable to generalise learning and so repeats a mistake if given a different context. Whilst we cannot see the cognitive damage we can infer there is damage by looking at the occupational performance.

7. **The environment.** The environment is viewed in its widest sense including the occupational behaviour context, objects, events, the physical environment, social groups and culture. Kielhofner suggests that the environment can be a powerful determinant of behaviour, saying it has an influence because of two processes. First, it 'affords' opportunities (or not). As an example here think of how a disabled person may be forced into inactivity because of physical barriers and mobility constraints. Secondly, the environment 'presses' for certain behaviours (e.g. the environment contains expectations and demands from others). A good example of this is how differently we behave when we are with different groups of people.

Application in occupational therapy

Occupational dysfunction is seen to occur when an individual has *difficulty choosing, organising or performing* his or her occupations. It is also a problem when occupational behaviour fails to provide quality of life or is insufficient to meet the demands of the environment. Kielhofner (1995, p. 183) spells this out in the following terms:

> When an individual's life demonstrates such loss, disruption of direction, lack of meaning or purpose that the person is unable to place himself or herself in a personal narrative which has possibilities and hope … then it may be said that the person is experiencing an occupational dysfunction. Moreover, society has a right to expect its members do their best to care for themselves and make reasonable contributions to the collective. When persons do not use their capacities in a reasonable way … we can also recognise occupational dysfunction.

The occupational therapist's role involves attempting to understand which component of the human system or environment is the most significant contributor to occupational dysfunction. To this end an enormous range of assessment tools and clinical reasoning protocols have been researched and developed (see Table 2.1).

Table 2.1 Assessment tools and the areas they assess based on the model of human occupation

	Volition	Habituation	Performance	Environment
Assessment Tools				
Assessment of Communication and Interaction Skills			X	
Assessment of Motor and Process Skills			X	
Assessment of Occupational Functioning	X	X	X	
The Interest Checklist	X			
NIH Activity Record	X	X		
Occupational Case Analysis Interview and Rating Scale	X	X	X	X
Occupational Performance History Interview	X	X	X	X
Occupational Questionnaire	X	X		
The Role Checklist	X	X		
Self Assessment of Occupational Functioning	X	X	X	X
Volitional Questionnaire	X			X
Worker Role Interview	X	X		X

The goal of treatment is to facilitate *change* though engaging the individual in action. For instance, we might enable someone to cope with a loss of a role and develop new occupational behaviours by introducing them to a new leisure pursuit. Kielhofner (1995, p. 256). explains that when therapy is successful it enables people to engage in occupational behaviour that continues their lives in a positive direction. 'The crux of all therapy is to get the patient to do something anew ... the onset of action begins the process of change.'

This process of change is not a linear process, however, it involves reorganising the whole system. For instance, if a person develops in their work skills (performance sub-system), the person's knowledge of his or her capacity is increased and confidence rises (volition). The person could then opt to change his or her occupational choices (volition) which results in new roles and work patterns (habituation). As the individual engages in the new work performance, skills increase (performance) and others around might comment positively (environment), which in turn encourages the person to take more risks (volition).

Evaluation

The strengths of this model are its sophisticated theoretical approach to understanding occupational behaviour whilst also being easy to apply practically (through using simple and relevant assessment tools). The model has many 'converts' who appreciate its use as a generic occupational therapy model suited to practice in many areas. Therapists seem to value it as a 'framework' or 'checklist' towards understanding occupational behaviour. A particular strength of the model is its in-depth exploration of both our volitional structure and the role of volition in initiating occupational behaviour.

Since its inception in the 1980s, the model of human occupation has generated a substantial and evolving research base. The research has occurred at three levels: (a) theoretical arguments have been validated or developed (research prompted Kielhofner *et al.* to revise the 1985 model to its current position in the 1995 version), (b) standard and published assessment tools have been developed (see Table 2.1), and (c) numerous clinical application studies have been described (e.g. Burton, 1989; Kaplan, 1986; Platts, 1993; Levine and Gitlin, 1993; Helfrich, Kielhofner and Mattingly, 1994).

Three major criticisms have been levelled at the model in the UK. First, some practitioners consider it does not travel well across the Atlantic. They say that American biases and assumptions means it has a limited application in the UK and that we should avoid unthinking, dogmatic adherence to it. Secondly, some of its conceptualisations are slightly weak or problematic. For instance, it can be criticised for being unduly focused on the individual with little exploration of social dynamics and environmental considerations. The performance sub-system in the 1985 version was particularly criticised as being insufficiently thought through. Also theorists like Mocellin (1996) criticise the focus on occupation, favouring the teaching and learning of skills (which brings about a sense of esteem, control, efficacy and self-determination) as the core concept. The third criticism which continues to be levelled at the model is that the 'jargon' and dense abstract ideas are difficult to follow. It takes a lot of time and effort to come to terms with the theoretical arguments (although arguably this is also a strength and the concepts do become easier with use).

To some extent, Kielhofner's 1995 revisions to the model answer these criticisms. Considerable detail has been added to the performance (now mind–brain–body performance) sub-system – aided largely by Fisher's (1994) AMPS research. Kielhofner and others have worked hard to emphasise the role of the environment and social/cultural meanings (i.e. different cultural practices). The model's research base, in particular regarding cross-cultural clinical applications, continues to develop.

The Occupational Performance Model

Key concepts

The Occupational Performance Model (developed by the Canadian Association of Occupational Therapists, 1991) can be summarised in terms of three main elements.

1. The model explores the interaction of **individuals** and their **occupations** which take place in a particular physical, cultural and social environment (see Figure 2.2).

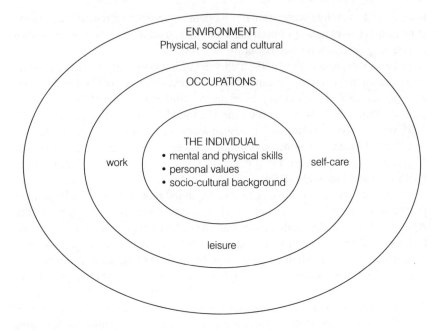

Figure 2.2 Interaction of individual, occupations and environment.

2. It retains a focus on **occupational performance** which takes into account the individual's developmental stages/needs, social roles and the environment.
3. It is a **client-centred** approach to practice, where the inter-dependent, collaborative relationship between client and therapist is stressed. Client-centred therapists attempt to view their clients holistically, value their individuality, respect their autonomy and allow them to make their own decisions (see Law, Baptiste and Mills, 1995).

The key ideas of the model are conceptualised using concentric elipses (see Figure 2.2) consisting of performance components, areas of occupational performance and the environment (see original figure in CAOT (1991), p. 17). The performance components are conceived in terms of their sociocultural background, mental and physical skills and the 'spiritual' (ethics and meanings rather than religion *per se*) values. Occupations are categorised as follows:

Productivity   paid–unpaid work
                  household management
                  play school
Leisure   quiet recreation

	active recreation
	socialising with others
Self-care	personal care (i.e. ADL)
	functional mobility
	community management (e.g. shopping)

Application in occupational therapy

The application of the Occupational Performance Model is best seen in the practical use of the Canadian Occupational Performance Measure (COPM) (Canadian
Association of Occupational Therapists, 1991) – an assessment which acts as a
clinical measure of the client's self-perception of occupational performance. The
COPM is a client-centred semi-structured interview and self-rating assessment
where the client identifies significant issues in daily activities which are causing
difficulty. The clients consider their full range of daily activities (self-care, productivity and leisure), and rate their importance, their perception of their performance and their level of satisfaction (scale of 1–10). After the occupational
therapy intervention, the assessment is repeated. The process allows the client and
therapist to have a numeric indication of changes perceived by the client.

Evaluation

The strength of this model is its client-centred approach and clearly articulated
focus on occupational performance. As such it is well in tune with our professional
philosophy and describes both the therapy process and our unique occupational
therapy focus.

The assessment has generated much interest in this country (helped by having
been piloted beyond Canadian borders in Britain, New Zealand and Greece). The
assessment is relatively straightforward to apply. It has the additional benefit that
it can be used to explain occupational therapy to both clients and team members.
Research on the application of the model and the COPM assessment (Law *et al.*,
1994; Toomey, Nicholson and Carswell, 1995; Waters, 1995) is still in its early
stages but looks promising.

The theoretical rationale underlying the model still needs to be developed further. Whilst the concept of client-centred practice has been well explained, the
other elements of the model could do with deeper exploration (rather than simply
asserting concepts and their relationship). Another criticism, suggested by some
practitioners is that the client-centred model is unrealistic since we can only strive
to be client-centred and never achieve it fully. Furthermore, this approach may
not be suitable for all clients (some may benefit from a more directive approach
and the COPM is more useful for clients with practical rather than emotional
problems).

Adaptation Through Occupation

Key concepts

In her book, *Models of Practice in Occupational Therapy*, Reed (1984) proposes an Adaptation through Occupation Model (initially presented in Sanderson and Reed, 1980). It arose in the context of the 1970s and 1980s where the models and theories used by occupational therapists tended to be borrowed from other fields. Reed aimed to articulate a clear view of occupational therapy and its outcomes. She set out to capture our unique focus and articulate how we conceptualise a person's problems.

Reed starts by emphasising how **'occupation'** is the unique organising concept of occupational therapy which is understood to give meaning to a person's life. It is seen as a dynamic process, changing in its form and components. Problems in occupation arise when (a) occupation becomes maladaptive, (b) when certain occupations hinder adaptation and (c) where a lack of occupation adversely affects health. Occupation itself is then used in treatment to facilitate adaptation.

The model largely consists of a concrete representation (see Figure 2.3) consisting of four main levels of analysis.

1. Occupation – which is divided into **self-maintenance**, **productivity** and **leisure**.
2. Five **performance areas** which are seen as necessary to carry out the occupations, i.e. motor, sensory, cognitive, intrapersonal and interpersonal skills.
3. The 'outcomes' of performing occupation are seen in terms of **actualisation**, **autonomy** and **accomplishment**.
4. The **environment** (biopsychological, physical and sociocultural) which is seen as determining the level of performance.

Application in occupational therapy

The goal of therapy according to this model is life satisfaction through occupations. Treatment is geared towards enabling people's occupations to meet their productivity, leisure and self-maintenance needs (e.g. ensuring they have the necessary skills).

Recently, the American Occupational Therapy Association (1994, p. 1047) published a generic outline and uniform terminology of our domain of concern to capture the essence of occupational therapy succinctly for others. Whilst this is not explicitly related to Reed's model, the similarities are striking, making it relevant for inclusion here. The framework described by the American Occupational Therapy Association (see Appendix V) divides our concern into:

Performance areas   activities of daily living; work and productive activities; and play or leisure

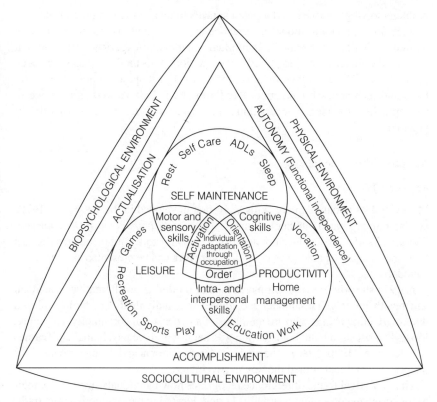

Figure 2.3 Reed's (from Reed, 1984) representation of adaptation through occupation.

Performance components sensori-motor, cognitive, psycho-social and psycho-logical

Performance context situations and factors that influence performance including temporal aspects (e.g. individual's age, health) and environment (physical, social, cultural)

The three areas are seen to interact, with functioning in the performance areas being the ultimate concern of occupational therapy. The associated Uniform Terminology Grid offers an interesting and detailed 'checklist' which therapists may find useful. Hansen and Atchinson (1993) go further and apply this grid to how conditions affect performance.

Evaluation

The main strength of this model is its relevance to occupational therapy given its focus on analysing occupations and occupational adaptation. The model offers a clear, reasonably simple representation of occupational therapy concerns and different levels of analysis. It succinctly encapsulates our holistic, client-centred, problem-solving approach and as such appeals to many practising therapists.

Arguably, it is not a 'model' of practice as it is limited in what it explains. In particular, it does not explain individual's behaviour/experience, nor does it explore the therapy process. Unlike the previous two models, it has not been particularly well researched or developed. Nor has it spawned any assessment tools and techniques for practice. Reed's model is best viewed as a device to conceptualise a person's occupational performance rather than as a guide for practice.

Adaptive Skills Model

Key concepts

Mosey's ideas about adaptive skills were first developed in the 1960s and 1970s and later incorporated into her volume *Psychosocial Components of Occupational Therapy*. Whilst Mosey does not describe a specific model of practice (as this is a term she equates to paradigm), chunks of her work can be presented as a theory or a model.

In 1974 she proposed the '**biopsychosocial model**' as an alternative to medical and health models. This model recognised that individuals are biological and thinking/feeling beings who are members of a wider social community. Arguably, Mosey's most significant contribution was her use of three psychological '**frames of reference**' (1970, 1986) – the analytical, acquisitional and developmental – for the practice of occupational therapy in psychiatry.

The **analytical** frame of reference recognises how individuals strive to get their needs (often unconscious) met and is largely located in the psychodynamic tradition. The **acquisitional** frame of reference stems from a cognitive-behavioural tradition and emphasises the acquisition of skills. The **developmental** frame (based on the work of Ayres and other developmental theorists) focuses on how adaptive skills are learned in a sequence.

In common with other developmental theorists, Mosey describes some basic principles which can be summarised in five points.

1. Development is the orderly progression of an individual through a series of complex, interacting stages.
2. An individual grows and learns in a sequential way – each gain provides the base for the next stage.
3. There are qualitatively different problems and opportunities that emerge at each stage – each of which need to be mastered.
4. Under stress or illness, individuals can regress to previous stages.
5. Treatment involves identifying the particular functioning level and providing experiences to facilitate step-by-step learning and adaptation (applied learning).

Application in occupational therapy

Mosey emphasised how occupational therapists are concerned with all aspects of

development and that we should apply our knowledge of 'normal' expectations to facilitate development in those impaired. She saw this being achieved by applying a *teaching–learning* process which included: (a) providing success experience that confirms stage learning, (b) encouraging safe exploration whilst practising skills and (c) providing opportunities for challenge.

Mosey's notion of adaptive skills offers us an account of both the sequence of development and how to intervene therapeutically. She outlines six (previously seven) areas of functioning or adaptive skills which are further divided into subskills. These sub-skills give us the specific ladder rungs or goals to use in the teaching/learning process.

The six **adaptive skills** can be summarised as (Mosey, 1986, pp. 416–442):

1. **Sensory integration skill** – the ability to co-ordinate vestibular, proprioceptive and tactile information for functional use.
2. **Cognitive skill** – the ability to organise sensory information for problem solving.
3. **Dyadic interaction skill** – the ability to engage in a variety of one-to-one relationships.
4. **Group interaction skill** – the ability to participate in a variety of groups.
5. **Self-identity skill** – the ability to perceive self as a relatively autonomous, acceptable person who has continuity over time.
6. **Sexual identity skill** – the ability to perceive one's sexual nature as good and participate in mutually enjoyable, long-term sexual relationships.

When treating a patient/client, it is not possible to work on all these areas at once, though a focus on one area usually prompts growth in another. Some occupational therapy units organise their programme around offering learning experiences related to one adaptive skill such as group interaction skill (see Table 2.2). In such a case, the process involved is one of: (a) identifying a newly referred patient's skills level, (b) slotting them in the appropriate level group (one that is both safe and offers challenges) and (c) facilitating 'higher' behaviours.

Table 2.2 Summary of group interaction sub-skills

Time period	Skills level	Interaction sub-skills
18 months–2 years	Parallel group level	Able to work alongside others in a group
2–4 years	Project group level	Minimally shares, competes and co-operates with prompting from the therapist
5–7 years	Egocentric-co-operative group level	Co-operative and competitive, experiments with group roles
9–12 years	Co-operative group level	Both positive and negative thoughts
15–18 years	Mature group level	Flexibility in taking on various roles within a hetereogeneous group

2.3 CASE ILLUSTRATIONS APPLYING OCCUPATIONAL THERAPY MODELS

Case illustration 2.1

Problem focus   Anxiety and limited meaningful occupations to structure each day
Model   The Model of Human Occupation

Jack is a 40-year-old man with a mild learning disability. He has been referred to an out-patient psychiatric service as he was having 'fits'/seizures which appeared to be anxiety related. The problem had become particularly severe over the last year when he regularly suffered severe shaking and went unconscious. He was hospitalised on several occasions but no organic cause was found.

Jack has a wife and three teenage daughters. He used to work in a tannery as a general dogsbody – a job which he enjoyed and which gave him a sense of purpose. He became unemployed 2 years ago. He is now highly anxious about his fits which results in him sitting in a chair all day long, doing nothing except waiting for the next fit to occur. For this reason, the psychiatrist referred Jack to the occupational therapist.

Occupational therapy assessment

The occupational therapist formed the following impression of Jack on giving him an initial interview:

> Jack is a shy, warm responsive man who is slightly slow in his understanding. He is overweight, unhealthy in appearance, rather sweaty and clearly anxious. Emotionally he is confused about everything: the interviews, investigations, hospitals, his fits and what was happening to his life. He dimly understands the fact that the occupational therapist works in a psychiatric unit, but finds it hard to understand that his fits are an emotional problem.
>
> He describes his typical day as 'doing nothing' [see Appendix II]. He has little in his life – no interests, little family involvement, no work – just a fear of when his next fit would occur where he would be required to go into hospital again. Jack's wife seems supportive in that she takes care of his basic self-care needs (keeping his house, feeding him, doing his laundry). His daughters tend to ignore him. Overall he appears to function at home like a lodger.

Applying the model of human occupation, the therapist made the following formulation:

Volition   Poor level of: interests, meaning in life, sense of personal causation. He feels out of control (related to his fits and loss of work).
Habituation   No productive roles or routines; sick role and passive habits adopted.
Performance   Low level of skill in all areas; some process skills problems related to using knowledge and transfer of learning.

Environment Wife seems supportive; hospital services now activated which are likely to be positive though care needs to be taken not to reinforce a sick role.

Treatment planning

The occupational therapist invited Jack to attend the occupational therapy department as an out-patient four mornings a week. This daily attendance aims to provide Jack with a structured, meaningful and active day in an effort to break the vicious cycle of his anxiety and inactivity. The daily contact also allows the therapist to assess Jack's potential further.

In discussion with the therapist, Jack completed a Modified Activity Record and an Interest Checklist self-rating scale (see Appendix I and II). On the basis of the information revealed, Jack and the therapist planned an activity programme which included a pottery session (with the focus on improving task skills) and a sports group (including football and swimming at the local swimming pool).

Problem area/treatment aims	Treatment method
Short term	
Habituation: break passive habits/routines.	*Environment* – day patient attendance for 4 mornings a week to give a meaningful structure to day.
Volition: re-activate meaningful activities and interests.	*Treatment activities* – (a) Pottery group. (b) Sports group. (c) Newspaper group.
Middle term	
Volition: develop sense of control and confidence in skills.	*Therapist approach* – allow more autonomy and decision making; give feedback (positive and constructively critical).
Habituation/performance: increase task performance skills and social interaction.	*Activity* – (a) Daily activity programme and gradually encourage the use of community facilities. (b) Cooking classes.
Long term	
Habituation: develop new productive roles (home work and reduce sick role).	*Therapist approach* – reduce dependence giving less support and expecting more from him.
Introduce new community-orientated habits.	*Activity* – cooking classes with 'homework'.
Resettlement to day centre for continued daily structure/stimulation.	*Environment* – more community activities and graded settlement to day centre.

Progress/evaluation

Jack attended the department conscientiously each morning and appeared to value his activity sessions (see Appendix III). He particularly enjoyed the pottery as he was learning new skills and he could give the end-products to his family. It was also an activity he would be able to continue long-term at a day centre. He also valued the swimming sessions as he had always wanted to learn to swim. After a few weeks of being accompanied Jack began to go to the pool independently or with his family. The activity of cooking was introduced at a later stage at Jack's request. He learned how to make three simple, tasty meals. He pleasantly surprised his family who gave him much praise and encouragement. He took on the role of cooking the dinner for his family once a week.

Over the course of 6 months Jack's condition improved considerably. He no longer had as many fits – and, importantly, when a fit occurred, he did not let it overtake his life. He no longer feared having a fit and felt if he did he would be all right. In terms of his daily life roles, his situation was dramatically altered through his occupational therapy programme. By the end of his treatment he had a much more active and satisfying life. His family relationships improved as he began to contribute to home life.

The one significant problem which occurred during his treatment was his reluctance to leave occupational therapy. The therapist recognised their error in encouraging too much dependence on their programme. Extra effort needed to be put into reducing his time and grading a discharge to the day centre.

Case illustration 2.2

Problem focus   Volitional narrative and replacing lost roles
Model   The Model of Human Occupation

Edna, 63 years old, was admitted to hospital with depression. It was triggered in part by the death of her husband, Vincent, last year. She felt she no longer had any meaning in her life. In hospital she was unmotivated to engage in treatment as she felt that nothing could change. However, the environment was supportive and she began to respond positively to the social contact around the ward.

Occupational therapy assessment

During the interview (using OPHI) Edna told the following story. She was born 63 years ago, the youngest child in a family of six children. Although they were poor, she had a happy childhood. Throughout her childhood she had one dream – to be a professional dancer. She loved dancing and with much determination she put in many hours of gruelling exercises and lessons in order to achieve her aim. When she was 17, she went to train in London and eventually joined a company. She was utterly committed to her profession and she remembers it as a very special time.

She gave up her dancing career to marry Vincent when she was 27 years old. Although she missed her dancing life dreadfully she felt she had to give it up in order to be a 'proper wife'. She maintained her routines of exercising and dancing for several hours each day, but this became something she did only for her own pleasure. Vincent and Edna had a full life together. They worked together managing their pet shop business. Socially, they were active theatre goers and played bridge and golf with friends. They had one son, Martin, whom they both adored.

Edna's middle years were basically happy and productive with the exception of two difficult periods of depression which occurred after the death of her mother and when Martin left home to go to University.

Fifteen years ago, Vincent suffered two severe strokes. He was left partially paralysed down his right side, with speech and perceptual problems and an unsteady, wide based gait. They sold their business, took early retirement and Edna devoted herself full-time to caring for her husband. Their leisure activities of golf and bridge playing were curtailed as Edna felt it was unfair to her husband for her to carry on doing these activities without him.

Over the years Vincent deteriorated in his functioning and Edna worked harder to care for him. She began to feel guilty/anxious every time she left him as Vincent played up in order to keep Edna by his side. Sometimes she arrived home from shopping or being with her friends, and would find Vincent balanced precariously on ladders or using dangerous power tools. Edna became more tired given the demands of caring for her husband and within a few years stopped having any sort of social life. Although she walked their dog daily, she was often too tired to carry out her dance exercises. She was stressed and exhausted but she was unable to attend to her own needs.

Edna was devastated when Vincent died. Not only had she lost her husband of 36 years, she had lost her main 'work' role. She also could not let go of a deep feeling of guilt that somehow she had failed him as his carer.

Edna felt unable to cope alone and moved into a small granny flat attached to her son Martin's house. She became increasingly dependent on him and the practical and emotional support he offered. When he had to go away on a month long business trip, Edna was unable to cope. Eleven months after Vincent's death, she was admitted to hospital with a severe depression. She felt she was a burden on her son and no longer wished to go on living (see Appendix IV for Role checklist, Values checklist and Interest checklist findings).

Treatment planning

Problem area/treatment aims	Treatment method
Short term	
Habituation: break passive habits/routines and activate new roles.	*Environment* – occupational therapy as out-patient.
Volition: develop personal causation (self awareness and knowledge of capacity).	*Treatment activities* – (a) One-to-one supportive counselling. (b) Movement to music class. (c) Photography group. (d) Creative group.

Middle term

Volition: develop sense of efficacy/control over self and outcomes.

Habituation: increase social contacts.

Goal setting in the community –
(a) At least 1 hour exercise dance each day.
(b) One productive outing daily, e.g. theatre, trip out, evening dance class, golf lessons, walk into town.
(c) Reactivate one social contact each week.

Long term

Habituation: develop new productive work and leisure roles.

(a) One-to-one counselling tailed off.
(b) Co-lead beginner's dance evening class.
(c) Re-join golf course.

Progress/evaluation

The focus of treatment was largely on trying to help Edna re-write or re-construct a new story for herself (volitional narrative): not as a dancer, not as a 'proper wife', not even as a 'carer' – but a story of an active person with lots of friends and hobbies. The climax of the treatment came in one session where she insisted she had nothing to give. The occupational therapist suggested a homework task to work out something. Edna came back the following session saying she could teach a beginner's dance class. She eventually achieved this. At the end of treatment she was able to re-claim enough of her previous self to construct a new life story for her future.

Case illustration 2.3

Problem focus   Resettlement in the community, emphasis on productivity
Model   Client-centred Occupational Performance Model

Sharon, 29 years old, has a long history of abusing drugs (including heroin), self-mutilation and crime (theft, shop lifting and making fraudulent social security claims). She has had several relationships with men who have abused her physically and has often lived rough (the first time when she ran away from home). She has spent the last 2 years being treated in a secure unit and is now preparing for discharge feeling motivated to begin a different life. The team have been closely involved with helping Sharon come off drugs and manage her 'out of control' feelings and behaviour. The team decided it was not time for a heavier occupational therapy input looking towards Sharon's re-integration back into the community. As this was a new stage of treatment, it was decided a new therapist should be involved who could relate to Sharon as she was now (rather than as someone who had shared her negative history).

Occupational therapy assessment

Over the course of several sessions the occupational therapist (using the Client-centred Occupational Performance Model) observed that Sharon presented inconsistently. At times she was full of bravado saying things like, 'I can't wait to get out of here away from all you screws' or 'I don't need your help I can look after myself'. At other times she seemed young and vulnerable, uncertain of how she was going to manage – scared she would simply return to her past life. As she once recognised, 'I only know how to be my past me. I don't know the future me. She's a stranger and she scares me'.

In order to enable Sharon to take control of her own life the therapist decided to use the COPM (determining a shared view of her problems/strengths and values/interests in relation to her future performance). With regard to self-care, Sharon described being unsure about how to make decisions and structure her day. She admitted to not taking care of her body before, but now she was trying to eat healthily and look after her appearance. In terms of *productivity*, Sharon's dream was to have a 'proper job' but she knew this was not going to happen easily as she had never worked before. Sharon thought her aunt might give her some work at her seaside cafe, which would supplement her social security benefit money. In terms of *leisure*, Sharon described having few hobbies outside her social life with her friends in the drug culture. In fact without the drug connection, she found social contact difficult. She enjoyed more solitary pursuits of watching videos and listening to music. She did, however, express an interest in learning to use the computer and play computer games.

Treatment planning

Treatment aims/outcomes	Treatment methods
Short term	
Leisure: to explore her interest in computer games and develop both skills and confidence in this area.	Daily practice on the computer in the OT department.
Productivity: to practice a range of domestic activities towards independent living.	Accompanied shopping in town plus cooking, budgeting, laundry, DIY sessions in the unit.
Long term	
Productivity: to investigate the possibility of computer classes; to investigate what computer games were available on the market and recommend three for the unit to buy; to approach Aunt Jean about the possibility of living and working with her.	Goals were negotiated and written down during a weekly one-to-one session.

Progress/evaluation

Sharon's rehabilitation took place over several months. Although she slipped back a number of times, she made good progress. She learned that she functioned best when busy and acknowledged the value of structuring her time. She quickly gained skill and confidence with computer work and took on the role of teaching others (including the occupational therapist!). She was also successful in researching and buying some new computer games for the unit. Sharon resolved to get a job and work to save up to buy her own computer.

On the domestic side, Sharon was not motivated to carry out any of the ordinary domestic rehabilitation activities. In these sessions she proved difficult and tended to be destructive, stirring up trouble with other group members. On review, the domestic programme was cancelled, although Sharon expressed an interest to learn how to cook Chinese food with a wok. This she did in a once a week one-to-one lunch cookery session (which included shopping for the ingredients) with the occupational therapist.

When Sharon eventually got the courage to contact her aunt she was offered part-time work at the cafe on a trial basis. This coincided with her discharge. She decided to move to temporary bed and breakfast accommodation at the seaside town. She agreed that moving to this new area would be slightly difficult in that she only knew her aunt. On the other hand, it would allow her a chance to start a completely new life.

Overall this treatment demonstrated the value of taking a client-centred approach where activities were chosen to be meaningful for Sharon. The occupational therapist would have liked her to become more involved with the domestic rehabilitation programme and with more social/group activities. However, the therapist recognised that it was important (for Sharon's motivation and esteem) to respond to her expressed preferences. Had the occupational therapist not done this Sharon might well have disengaged from treatment and not faced the stress/demands of changing her life.

Case illustration 2.4

Problem focus   Lack of balance in occupations
Model   Adaptation through Occupation Model

Bill, 78 years old, is an ex-army major. After the war, he became a property developer, specialising in large-scale developments (e.g. old manor houses). Bill retired 10 years ago intending to travel with his wife, but this proved impossible when she developed dementia. Bill eventually took on a full-time carer role as his wife was dependent on him for all aspects of her ADL. Lately Bill has become exhausted and stressed with his caring role, and has developed angina. He was referred to a community occupational therapist for advice on conserving his resources and some stress management.

Occupational therapy assessment

Bill presented as a 'gentleman' who was very concerned and anxious about his wife. He tended to do everything for her – both personal care and taking over all domestic responsibilities – and he constantly worried if he was doing things correctly. The interview revealed he has taken these roles so much to heart that he no longer had any time for himself.

The therapist conceptualised Bill's situation in the following way:

> Bill's main problem appears to be a lack of balance in his occupations. His complete focus on 'productivity' (related to home management and his caring role) gives him a sense of accomplishment and he values the role of caring for his wife (related to sociocultural norms). However, his own leisure and self-maintenance has suffered which has negatively impacted on his health and his level of general satisfaction (actualisation).

The therapist advised Bill he needed to take some time out to rest and care for himself, as well as to re-engage in leisure occupations for both enjoyment and 'renewal'. The primary treatment aim concerned developing a balance of occupations such that actualisation, autonomy and achievement were attained.

Progress/evaluation

Initially Bill was reluctant to ease off on his domestic/caring roles as he was anxious about how his wife would manage. With the help of the occupational therapist he began to see the link between his angina, stress and lack of balance in occupations. He eventually saw the logic of bringing in some outside domestic and nursing help. The occupational therapist also advised him on how to manage his wife's ADL. It emerged from an ADL assessment carried out on his wife, that she was more able than he had imagined. Bill learned to stand back a bit more though this was difficult for him and he often lapsed into doing things for his wife. The therapist reasoned that it gave Bill a sense of accomplishment and satisfaction.

Bill was encouraged to take up some old hobbies and meet up with some friends at a club. With the therapist's prompting, he agreed the goal that he would take one trip abroad each year without his wife. On the day of his discharge, Bill proudly showed the therapist a return air ticket for a holiday in Cyprus that he had just bought.

Case illustration 2.5

Problem focus   Process of teaching and learning group interaction skills
Model   Adaptive Skills (Developmental) Model

Willis, 30 years old, was an in-patient in a psychiatric hospital with a diagnosis of schizophrenia. His disorder resulted in him being withdrawn, self-absorbed and he occasionally made bizarre comments which affected his ability to relate to others.

Occupational therapy assessment

The occupational therapist assessed Willis' task performance and group interaction skills during a cooking group and in other task activities. The therapist observed that Willis seemed unaware of other people's needs and appeared to find it difficult to share (for instance, he took over the cooker area and only moved when prompted). He only interacted with the therapist when a direct question was asked, otherwise he remained withdrawn. The occupational therapist considered he was functioning developmentally at a low project group level.

Treatment planning

Willis' difficulty in group interaction prompted a referral to the Project Group. The Project Group was a group that was already established and consisted of seven other patients functioning at or marginally below project group interaction level. The group would meet daily for an hour to engage in a mixture of activities. The treatment programme described below shows how the art activity of collage was graded and adapted.

Progress/evaluation

1. *Early-level project group experience.* Willis was introduced to the group and joined their activity, which took place around one table. Each patient was asked to make his or her own individual collage, from cutting out pictures of food from magazines and sticking them onto a sheet of paper. At the end the occupational therapist encouraged the group members to be aware of each other and work together more, by asking them to arrange each individual's sheet with the others, on a larger poster. Willis found the latter task of working with the whole group more difficult, so he remained more passive.
2. *Medium-level project group experience.* After a few sessions similar to the above, the occupational therapist encouraged Willis and the others to make a collage in pairs, requiring them to minimally share and interact with at least one other person. Willis enjoyed this and was also able to work a bit with the group as a whole, as they discussed how to arrange the pictures.
3. *Advanced-level project group experience.* On a later occasion the occupational therapist encouraged the group to make a collage as a whole. Individuals first collected their own pile of 'rubbish', such as leaves or empty matchboxes. These were then placed all together in a pile. The group then stuck the bits randomly onto a large card. Willis was given the responsibility at the end to spray the collage an attractive gold colour. At this level of group working the therapist attempted to further group sharing and awareness of others by promoting discussion and also by reducing the amount of glue and scissors available.

2.4 OTHER RELEVANT THEORIES

Occupational behaviour theory

Mary Reilly developed the concept of occupational behaviour as the key occupational therapy domain of concern. Her work, dating back to the 1940s, is arguably the most significant early influence on the evolution of our profession. She developed her theory throughout the 1960s and 1970s at the University of Southern California, leading a group of graduate students and colleagues (including Matsutsuyu, Florey, Kielhofner and Takata amongst others).

From her earliest work, Reilly emphasised the 'occupation' in occupational therapy. She believed the main aim of occupational therapy was to promote life satisfaction through engaging in life role tasks. She emphasised that treatment should address dysfunctions (i.e. in coping with play, work and school situations). Reilly was one of the first to articulate a unique body of occupational therapy knowledge which has become a foundation for subsequent theories (e.g. the Model of Human Occupation).

The occupational behaviour theory can be summarised as five key points.

- Central focus on occupation recognising how individuals are intrinsically motivated to engage in occupation.
- Any therapy should pivot on looking at expectations of a person's life roles and associated tasks which also need to be seen in the context of a developmental continuum.
- Children's play is critical for developing the adaptive skills necessary to be competent in later adult roles.
- Work/play roles have an organising influence and having a balanced experience of work, play and self-maintenance is important.
- The environment is important for supporting or impeding adaptation (based on a 'systems' view).

Cognitive Disabilities Model

Claudia Allen's (1985) Cognitive Disabilities Model stands out from other occupational therapy models in its philosophy as it tends to emphasise a person's limitations rather than their potential. Its key premise is that neurological problems produce cognitive limitations (e.g. difficulty in learning), which in turn results in reduced performance. The model was originally developed as an approach to treating chronic psychiatric patients, but since has developed to be used for other groups (such as people with learning disabilities and those suffering from dementia).

The model proposes a continuum of function and dysfunction divided into six cognitive levels.

Level 1 This level represents profound cognitive disability where the person is conscious but largely unaware of other people/environment.

Level 2 Here, individuals can follow very simple instructions; they often wander or pace aimlessly and are only partially aware of the environment.

Level 3 At this level individuals can begin to carry out manual actions and use physical objects (e.g. they can carry out repetitive self-care tasks).

Level 4 Individuals at this level are beginning to be purposeful and goal directed; with help they can complete concrete tasks.

Level 5 People at this level show more flexibility and can attend to all elements in their environment. New learning can occur but problems are still apparent, e.g. anticipating or planning events and abstract thinking are still difficult to do.

Level 6 Individuals at this level function well. They can pre-plan actions, follow instructions, consider hypothetical possibilities and understand abstract concepts.

The model provides detailed procedures for assessing patients (by observing their task performance using the Allen Cognitive Level test amongst other assessments). It also offers in-depth guidelines for analysing and structuring activities which are matched to the relevant level of cognitive function. Allen stresses the need to acknowledge and work within permanent limitations of the patient's capacity.

Sensory Integration Model

Jean Ayres developed the Sensory Integration Model using her observations that children with learning disabilities found it difficult to interpret sensory information (from their bodies and the environment) and that these difficulties were associated with broader developmental delay. She drew on a neuroscience theoretical base plus applied normal development studies to formulate the three basic principles underlying sensory integration, i.e.

1. Early vestibular, tactile and proprioceptive experiences are important in personality development.
2. Perceptual processes are crucial for the individual to adapt to the human and non-human environment.
3. Carefully chosen motor and sensory activities can be effective therapy for those with deficits in their integration.

She identified four basic sensory integration disorders: (a) problem with processing vestibular–proprioceptive sensation, (b) problem with processing tactile and proprioceptive information, (c) difficulty responding to sensations, and (d) dyspraxia and clumsiness. To assess these problems the therapist can use both informal procedures and a formalised battery of tests (Sensory Integration and Praxis tests). Treatment involves selecting appropriate experiences to stimulate the child's deficit areas. Play activities are commonly used to encourage the child to engage in the relevant sensory motor behaviours. (For a more detailed account of sensory integration theory and practice, see Fisher, Murray and Bundy, 1991.)

The sensory integration model has been primarily applied in the US, but there are practitioners in the UK who have undertaken relevant specialist training (see Fairgrieve, 1996). Ayres was a prolific writer and followers of this tradition continue to publish their research in many journals.

Occupational science

The new field of occupational science is not a model of occupational therapy but it does promise to become a relevant theory and research base for the profession. It has grown out of the work of Larson, Clark, Yerxa and others in the US, and has now evolved its own journal (*Journal of Occupational Science Australia*). It is being presented as a new 'social science' designed to study: humans as occupational beings, the purpose of occupation in survival and health, and how humans realise a sense of meaning through activity.

The main ideas are encapsulated in the following quote:

> Occupational science will study the person's experience of engagement in occupation recognising that observing behaviour is not sufficient for understanding occupation. The organisation and balance of occupations in daily life and how these relate to adaptation, life satisfaction and social expectations will be central issues as will timing, planning and anticipation. Occupational science will seek to learn more about intrinsic motivation and the drive for effectance. Finally it will need to be true to its humanistic roots by preserving human complexity, diversity and dignity. (Yerxa *et al.* 1990, cited in Hagedorn, 1995, p. 91.)

The field of occupational science has led to a certain amount of debate (see the 1991 issues of *American Journal of Occupational Therapy*) between those who feel it is a distinct science separate from occupational therapy and those who feel it is part of our professional theoretical base. It will be interesting to see how it evolves over the next decade.

CONCLUSION

The models and theory explored in this chapter give us our unique occupational therapy 'gaze'. The chapter has shown how models can act as our spectacles through which we view both the patient/client and the treatment process. Whilst the models differ slightly in how they conceptualise function/dysfunction, it is no accident that the models share a preoccupation with occupation, activity, adaptation, performance skills and development. Arguably, without such a unifying, theoretical base, we cannot call ourselves a profession.

The following chapter continues to explore the role of theory but shifts the focus to looking at theories drawn from other disciplines (i.e. psychology). Such theory offers us our treatment methods and tools.

Discussion questions

1. Why do we need occupational therapy models?
2. Compare and contrast any two occupational therapy models.
3. What is meant by the terms theory, model and approach?
4. Take one occupational therapy model and analyse its strengths and weaknesses.
5. Consider Case illustration 2.1. How would Jack's treatment have been altered by applying different models of practice?
6. Should our profession draw on many different generic as well as occupational therapy models of practice?

Psychological theories and approaches

The field of psychology offers us different theories which help us to understand and explain human behaviour and experience. Consider, for example, the case of Joe, a retired gentleman who has a special hobby collecting stamps. A **behaviourally** orientated psychologist might explain Joe's hobby as Joe modelling on his father who had collected stamps and encouraged his interest. A **psychodynamically** inclined psychologist might suggest Joe is a 'collector' and given he enjoys the detailed, obsessional work involved in cataloguing the stamps, he could be an 'anal personality' type. A **humanistic** psychologist, on the other hand, might focus on how Joe takes pleasure in stamp collecting and the status that goes along with it, and so he chooses to do it. A **sociologically** inclined psychologist would instead point to how Joe has selected a hobby suited to an intelligent, middle class, middle-aged man looking for good financial investment in our Western culture. Each of these theories/perspectives offer us potential insights and, as such, act as an *analytical tool* towards understanding Joe's behaviour.

Beyond being a tool, however, each theory also carries with it an *implication for practice* – more specifically, implications for treatment. Take the case of Betty. She is a woman who is suffering from agoraphobia (fear of going outside). **Cognitive-behavioural** therapists are likely to see her problem in terms of a 'habit' of negative thinking and avoidance behaviour, exacerbating her anxiety spiral. They would get her gradually to face going outside. **Psychodynamic** therapists would seek to look underneath Betty's fear and explore her unconscious desires. The symbolic meaning of going outside would be sought in therapy, in order to help her gain insight into her inner conflicts. **Humanists** would focus on her self-image as someone who cannot cope outside. They would employ counselling and other techniques to enable her to feel more confident and in control of her life. The therapists favouring more **social explanations** might point to the gender dimension and ask why most agoraphobics in our society are women. A women's support group might be recommended as a suitable treatment. Thus,

Betty's *treatment depends entirely on which theoretical perspective is adopted by her therapist.*

In the first section of this chapter, we will explore the use of three theoretical frameworks arising from the field of psychology, i.e. the psychodynamic, behavioural and humanistic approaches. A fourth 'social' perspective (really an amalgamation of several social psychology/sociology theories) will be offered as a contrast. I will first review the main ideas of each approach, then discuss, in turn, the way these ideas have been applied in occupational therapy. In the second section, the contrast between the theories will be illustrated by using three different case examples which apply the theory in practice. The concluding section will offer a wider discussion and evaluation of the approaches.

3.1 FOUR PSYCHOLOGICAL APPROACHES

The psychodynamic approach

Key concepts

The psychodynamic approach is based on the ideas of Freud's psychoanalytic theory and later developed by many subsequent theorists/therapists. The approach can be summarised in terms of two core ideas: (a) the importance of childhood experience and relationships on development, and (b) the significance of the unconscious.

1. **Role of development.** First, psychodynamic theorists emphasise the idea that early childhood development and experience influences adult personality. In Freud's view, a child is seen to move through a developmental sequence of stages of **psychosexual development** (oral, anal, phallic, latency, genital). Childhood experience through these stages was seen to affect later adulthood in that feelings could be transferred into adult relationships. Thus, if a child experiences certain traumas (or is deprived or is overgratified) at any stage, he/she can become 'fixated' (i.e. stuck) at that stage. For example, a person who is dependent and 'needy' as an adult, could be fixated in the oral stage, mirroring a baby's need for nurturing.
2. **Significance of the unconscious.** The second core idea is the existence of a dynamic, conflicted unconscious. Freud conceptualised humans as having three unconscious aspects of self: the **id** (driven by primitive biological needs and impulses), the **ego** (the logical, thinking self which mediates demands of the id and **super-ego**) and the super-ego (the moral conscience where the values of parents/society are adopted). The balance of these three aspects (formed in childhood) are seen to influence an adult's personality in that problems arise when one part is over controlling or under active (e.g. an over controlling super-ego produces excessive guilt; insufficient super-ego results in psychopathic behaviour). Beyond these three aspects, the unconscious is seen as a

repository of powerful emotions/needs at war with each other. The conflicts and anxieties generated by this war are unconsciously 'handled' by developing defence mechanisms such as repression, projection and sublimation.

A *social dimension*

Much of Freud's original psychoanalytic theory has been developed and considerably modified by many subsequent theories (hence we use the term *psychodynamic*) over the last 50 years. For instance, his focus of sexuality has been marginalised in favour of a more social interactionist line. Early childhood experiences are still seen as important – but instead of sexual development, modern day psychoanalysis emphasise the quality of the **parent–baby relationship**. In object relations theory, for example, the child's early relationships are seen as playing a critical role in developing the child's ability to relate to others as this is where the child learns to love, trust and interact mutually with others. When early positive bonding is missing or relationships are distorted in some way, the child is likely to have problematic relationships in the future. Bowlby (1971, 1975) was a psychoanalyst who studied attachment theory and separation anxiety. Other psychologists (e.g. Rutter, 1995) took up these ideas and showed that difficulties in relating to others seem to follow from early institutionalisation, lack of consistent care and/or distorted, tense family relationships.

Erikson (1977) is one theorist who has developed a more social dimension of psychoanalytic theory. He identifies how the identity/ego develops and changes throughout life. He identifies eight life cycle stages. He characterises each stage in terms of a developmental conflict which needs to be resolved which enables the ego to be strengthened and a special quality to develop. Importantly, each stage is set in both a biological and social/cultural context. For instance, the combination of physical ageing and society's negative attitudes to old age may well precipitate despair in later years.

The work of Bion (1961), an influential group analyst, provides another example of a more social orientation. He applied psychoanalytic ideas to the group situation. He initiated the idea of viewing a group as a whole, not as simply a collection of individuals. Moreover, he considered that two agendas operate in groups – an overt, conscious agenda and a hidden agenda consisting of unconscious intra-group tensions and emotions.

THEORY INTO PRACTICE

Defensive manoeuvres in a group – the application of psychodynamic ideas to a group context

Bion's ideas of overt and hidden agendas can be illustrated by the following example of what occurred in one ward group. The group was experiencing a fair amount of interpersonal tensions – though much of it remained unexpressed (it felt too unsafe to be honest). Mostly, the group members avoided personal discussion by talking about issues outside the ward. In particular, a couple of members were allowed to intellectualise at length. In one meeting, one member challenged the way they were monopolising the discussion with their intellectualising. He was then roundly criticised by other members who felt he was insufficiently involved in and committed to the ward activities.

Some possible interpretations of the group's hidden agenda are as follows. (a) The group avoided dealing with their interpersonal conflicts by colluding with intellectualised discussion about outside issues (i.e. the discussion was a defensive manoeuvre). (b) The group turned against and scapegoated the member who challenged the defensive strategy. (c) Scapegoating the member carried with it two pay-offs: it united the group and it ensured that defensive avoidance was maintained, thus enabling the group to continue to avoid looking at their own material. (d) The criticism levelled at the one member about insufficient commitment may well have been a product of the members' own projections.

The psychodynamic treatment approach

The psychodynamic treatment approach involves two stages: to express unconscious feelings, then explore and 'work through' conflicts (e.g. by gaining insight and so strengthening the ego). A variety of treatment methods are used. Classical psychoanalysis usually involves years of 'being on the couch' where the analyst listens to the patients' stories and tries to uncover unconscious meanings through using techniques such as dream interpretation and word association. Psychodynamic therapists can adopt a broader range of treatment methods encompassed under the banner of '**psychotherapy**'. Psychotherapy can occur in a group or one-to-one situation and largely involves expressing/exploring dynamics (i.e. unconscious processes, feelings and transferences) of relationships.

THEORY INTO PRACTICE

Insights arising from a psychodrama session

Carole used a psychodrama session to explore her ambivalent feelings about becoming a mother. She was frightened she was going to abuse her baby. In a psychodramatic construction (and with the support of group members) she acted out her worst nightmare where she threw the baby against a wall. The director then guided her to become the baby and (with someone else playing Carole) enter into a dialogue with her. Through this role reversal Carole was able to acknowledge, for the first time, feelings about her own abusive mother. With the group's help she realised she did not have to recreate what happened to her with her own children. The session ended with the group holding and rocking Carole. She began to explore what it meant to be nurtured and nurturing. The overall psychodrama experience was intense, emotional and deeply moving.

Psychodynamic approach applied to occupational therapy

Occupational therapists do not 'do' psychoanalysis. We can, however, draw on psychodynamic ideas, for instance:

1. We focus on the importance of **interpersonal relationships** in therapy (between therapist and patient and between patients). We explore the transferences and interactions which occur within therapy to help patients/clients understand themselves better. We also use group situations to explore wider relationship dynamics.
2. We recognise the potential **power of the unconscious** and peoples' use of defence mechanisms when they are in pain or conflict.
3. We recognise the importance of **ego boundaries** and how that impacts on self-identity and relationships.
4. We exploit the symbolic and **projective potential of activities** to encourage the expression and exploration of feelings, for instance in our use of projective art.

Gail and Jay Fidler were influential in the 1960s in bringing this psychodynamic approach into occupational therapy. Like other psychoanalytical therapists, they stressed the role of the unconscious and **object relations** in influencing behaviour. Their theory and practice emphasised three other key processes.

1. They argued that communication is the essence of occupational therapy. They saw the inability to communicate effectively as the key psychiatric disability. Thus, in occupational therapy, the process and end-product of activities are designed to facilitate individuals to communicate thoughts/feelings which they cannot express at a verbal level.
2. They then stressed the importance of interpersonal relationships in therapy. In the treatment process both the patient–therapist relationship and the patients interactions in a group are considered of central significance (e.g. for strengthening the ego and for reality testing).
3. They further emphasised the symbolic potential of activities to allow the exploration of conflicts. Activities are seen as useful in dealing with self-concept; sexual identity; infantile, oral and anal needs; dependency; hostility and reality testing (Fidler and Fidler, 1963).

THEORY INTO PRACTICE

Applying psychodynamic concepts in occupational therapy
Consider the following treatment example of how clay work was used projectively in a psychotherapy–playtherapy session with a disturbed 9-year-old girl called Tracy.

Therapists plan of session
Aims – Projective clay work to:

1. Provide an opportunity for Tracy to regress symbolically.

2. Offer an opportunity for her to express and explore her feelings (in particular anger) towards her family.
3. Provide a safe environment to experience constructive and destructive action.

Method
1. Tracy to create each family member in clay.
2. Offer time for Tracy to express what she is trying to represent.
3. Through play, Tracy to represent 'how the family is' and 'how she wishes it to be'

Therapist's account of the session
Tracy started by creating her father – a special, much loved figure; then stepmother (loathed 'wicked witch'); and then the new baby (loathed interloper). Using the figure of herself she 'kicked' her stepmother around and tore the baby to bits. She then had her father apologise to her for marrying 'that awful woman' and the two of them settled down to 'live happily ever after'. After encouraging some exploration of this need I challenged Tracy's claim that that was how she wanted it to be. She then slowly remade the stepmother piece, and placed her parents and herself into a close idealised family (without the baby!).

Significant themes
Sibling rivalry and competition with stepmother for father's love emerge clearly. Tracy has used the play session powerfully to express and act out her needs. By expressing the conflicts Tracy is beginning to understand her 'bad' behaviour at home.

The cognitive-behavioural approach

Key concepts

The cognitive-behavioural approach focuses on **learning** as the key to development and socialisation. This perspective maintains that children are born a 'blank slate' and are required to learn virtually everything – to talk, read, be toilet trained, study, play, socialise, etc.

According to behaviourists, learning occurs through the stimulation and rewards available in the environment. We routinely praise, encourage, reward, punish and even ignore children to change or develop their behaviour. Take for example how Colin's father taught 6-year-old Colin how to ride a bicycle. Colin had had a bad accident when he first tried to ride a two wheeler – now he was frightened of it, saying he did not want to learn and he would stick to his tricycle. Colin's father set out to teach him. First, he helped Colin associate bicycling with fun and safety by holding on to him whilst playfully wheeling him around. He gradually introduced the idea of letting go for a few seconds and using a lot of praise when Colin successfully rode by himself. Once Colin could ride by himself, his father rode another bicycle alongside to act as both a model and as an encourager. All of these ideas are based on scientifically researched, behavioural techniques, i.e. classical/operant conditioning, cognitive-behavioural theory and social learning theory, each of which is described below.

Traditional behaviourism

Classical conditioning consists of learning by *association*. For instance, it is a common experience to suddenly experience tooth pain on hearing a drill. As another example, consider the case of Bill who is no longer able to bear the smell of whiskey since he associates it with a previous occasion when he overindulged and was sick.

With operant conditioning learning occurs in three ways: (a) we repeat behaviours when they are rewarded (**positive reinforcement**), (b) learning can occur by removing aversive stimuli (**negative reinforcement**) and (c) learning can occur by applying a negative or removing a positive stimulus (**punishment**) – however, whilst punishment can be effective for a while, research has shown that the undesired behaviour will come back if nothing more positive replaces it. Thus if a parent criticises a child (punishment) for interrupting a conversation, the child may well stop interrupting for a while. However, unless children are taught what else to do, they will return to interrupting (not least because criticism may be better than no attention at all!). In other words, operant conditioning states that if we want to change the way someone behaves, we need to replace it by reinforcing new, desired behaviours.

Cognitive-behavioural theory

Traditional behaviourism tends only to focus on observable behaviour and processes (stimulus–response) and ignores internal processes such as thinking/emotions. This is a major weakness which more recent cognitive-behavioural theory attempts to redress. By recognising *thinking* and *motivation*, cognitive-behaviourism is much more able to explain complex learning such as learning how to talk. It also explains how we pick up beliefs and attitudes (like prejudice) better than more traditional models/theories.

Cognitive behaviourism emphasises the point that thinking, motivation and the social context all play a significant role in learning. Take, for example, the situation where you are trying to teach Dorothy how to use a video camera. If she is going to learn effectively, she needs first to want to learn, then to respect your ability as a teacher. In terms of teaching the skill, it would not be sufficient to teach her by rewarding her each time she accidentally touches the correct button. Instead, you would need to teach the logic of each operation.

Some cognitive behaviourists go beyond the idea that thinking is a part of learning and assert that *thinking patterns themselves affect behaviour*. A classic example is Susan who is phobic about exams. On having to face an exam, she gets trapped in a negative spiral of thinking. She starts by thinking, 'I can't cope with exams … I'm no good at them … I always fail … I'm going to fail this one … I can feel myself getting panicky … I won't be able to control it …'. She soon talks herself into a full blown panic attack. Therapists who adopt this theory say that

Susan's behaviour will only change by changing the pattern of her negative thoughts (see the Theory into Practice box on p. 53 on applying behavioural concepts in occupational therapy).

A social dimension

Social learning theory is a particular approach which comes under the banner of cognitive behaviourism. It proposes that learning occurs in a social context through imitation and modelling on others. The best way to learn to ski, for example, is to model on the instructor's demonstration. Moreover, we not only copy but we select what we want to model on and we can learn vicariously through others – be it friends, parents, off the TV, etc. We do not copy all the behaviour we observe, so there must be an element of thinking and selecting behaviours we wish to reproduce. Bandura suggests that the behaviours we choose to imitate will be ones where we anticipate a positive consequence (which leads us back to conditioning).

THEORY INTO PRACTICE

Current research demonstrating the complex interaction of cognitive and social factors involved with alcoholism

There is heated debate in the literature about the validity of the biological disease model for alcoholism which suggests addiction is a result of either brain chemical imbalances or genetic inheritance (Toates, 1996). Other research demonstrates the need to consider wider cognitive and social factors. Cox and Klinger (1988) offer a model of alcohol consumption which suggests people decide to drink on the basis of weighing up positive consequences as people with alcohol problems may believe that taking a drink will make them more sociable, relaxed, confident, etc. Other research, such as Perri (1985), demonstrates a correlation between a person being able to give up drinking and their ability to find alternative behaviour patterns (e.g. new hobbies). Alexander (1990) focuses more on the role of the addict's personality combined with cultural pressures. Alexander writes '... the mind-numbing addict culture is more bearable than isolation. Chronic intoxication, although unhealthy and boring, can provide distraction from a corrosive preoccupation with failure' (1990, p. 39).

The cognitive-behavioural treatment approach

Behavioural methods of treatment have been widely applied in mental health and in teaching people skills. Some specific behavioural techniques are:

- **Systematic desensitisation** – where a person is gradually introduced into a feared stimulus (e.g. with agoraphobia the person has progressive goals of walking to the front gate, then down the road 50 m, 100 m ...).

- **Token economy** – where tangible rewards (e.g. sweets, tokens, stars) are systematically given to increase positive behaviours.
- **Chaining or backward chaining** – where skills are taught in a linked sequence (e.g. breaking learning into small steps like teaching a child to pull up socks, then put them on).

Cognitive therapy is commonly used in anxiety management programmes. Clark (1986) proposed a cognitive approach to panic which involved the following sequence of events. First, the individual becomes apprehensive which results in autonomic nervous system responses such as increased heart rate and hyperventilation. These are then in turn interpreted as 'catastrophic' which increases the panic. Cognitive therapists advocate various strategies which focus on the anxious individual's beliefs. These strategies include trying to get him or her to realise that: (a) attending to bodily sensations can lead to greater anxiety, (b) bodily symptoms can be controlled and (c) catastrophic consequences (like a heart attack) do not occur. In researching the effectiveness of such an approach, Clark *et al.* (1994) compared the outcomes of cognitive therapy, relaxation training and the use of the drug imipramine. Cognitive therapy emerged as more effective (both after the therapy and 15 months later).

The cognitive-behavioural approach applied to occupational therapy

Occupational therapists draw widely on behavioural principles. We routinely apply them unconsciously/automatically (e.g. in our use of rewarding with praise or when we give someone 'feedback'). We consciously and systematically *apply behavioural principles* when teaching patients/clients new skills and behaviours. Here, for instance, we might employ 'backward chaining methods' to teach a child to dress or systematic desensitisation as part of an anxiety management programme.

The application of cognitive-behavioural theory has more or less replaced the more mechanistic, traditional behaviourism in occupational therapy. We would, for example, be more likely to see occupational therapists exploiting group treatment situations (such as assertiveness training or anxiety management groups which offer opportunities for social learning) rather than token economy programmes. Mosey's work in defining the dimensions of the occupational therapy **teaching–learning process** is a good illustration of the need to consider wider motivational and social factors – especially the relationships between the teacher and the learner. As she states, 'A therapist can only help a client want to learn through the design of appropriate learning situations' (Mosey, 1986, p. 218).

THEORY INTO PRACTICE

Applying behavioural concepts in occupational therapy

Occupational therapists commonly use the cognitive-behavioural approach when teaching stress management techniques (in a group or on an individual basis). Consider the following treatment in which Susan learned to manage her exam phobia.

Stage 1   Education: Susan was advised about the nature of anxiety and how a certain amount was necessary for peak performance.

Stage 2   Cognitive restructuring: Susan was first taught to think differently about her anxiety, e.g. to look on it as a 'potentially helpful friend' and not 'an out of control enemy'. Second, she rehearsed a new sequence of more positive thinking like, 'I am not going to fail, I know I can do it, I have done it in practice. I have worked hard and I want to demonstrate my knowledge'. Susan was then given some homework which involved chanting this sequence every time she caught herself thinking about exams negatively.

Stage 3   Relaxation: Susan learned a range of relaxation techniques. She had to think through which would be more suitable for her in different situations.

Stage 4   Systematic desensitisation: Susan eventually had to face up to the practical side of actually sitting in an exam room under exam conditions. In order to prepare for this Susan and her therapist drew up a plan of action – breaking down the task into more manageable chunks (which included built in rewards and the application of relaxation techniques). (a) Susan first was to sit down in her empty college exam hall comfortably. (b) She was then to manage (successfully) a prepared mock exam question her tutor supplied. (c) She would then move on to complete (successfully) a full mock exam.

The humanistic approach

Key concepts

The humanistic (sometimes called phenomenological) perspective developed in the 1950s as a reaction to the determinism of the psychodynamic approach and the reductionism of the behaviourist approach. It operates both as an existential philosophy (e.g. asking about the meaning of life) and as an approach to therapy. Different theorists and therapists who operate within this perspective often offer different accounts of human development; however, they all share similar preoccupations with the individual, self-identity, freedom/autonomy and subjective meanings/needs.

Sense of self

Central to the humanistic approach is the **concept of 'self'**. Humanists assert that each of us is unique and made up of our own individual thoughts, feelings, behaviours, attitudes, bodies, past experiences, etc. Thus we have a self-awareness, a self-identity, a sense of ourselves as continuing – there is only one of us. We have a sense of 'I'. Importantly, we also have the capacity to **reflect** on our experience of being that individual. Carl Rogers (1961), arguably the most famous humanistic therapist, has written much about self-concept. He argues that the way we perceive ourselves affects the way we experience and respond to events. The greater the congruence between what he called our 'actual self' (i.e. how we are) and our 'ideal' self (i.e. how we would like to be), the better adjusted we are.

Autonomy

We also have a sense of our own power and **agency**. We can do things to, and produce an effect on, others and our environment. I can cook a meal. I can make someone else feel happy. I can put out a fire. Along with the capacity to do, I can choose to do. I can even choose to die. To a greater or lesser degree, we are free agents – we have freedom of choice. As Glover puts it, we are who we are because we want to be that way, 'To varying degrees we take charge of our lives. Through controlling our actions by our own plans, we become active rather than passive ... Consciously shaping our own characteristics is self-creation' (Glover, 1988, as cited in Stevens, 1991, p. 14).

Focus on subjective experience

Whilst psychodynamic therapists work with unconscious needs, humanistic therapists home in on conscious experience and **subjective meanings** (beliefs, feelings, needs, motivations). Abraham Maslow (1954), another theorist in this genre focuses on motivation. He conceptualises motives in terms of a hierarchy of needs, i.e. physiological, safety, love/belonging, esteem, cognitive/aesthetic and then finally self-actualisation. As each lower order need is met, we perceive and are challenged by the next one.

A social dimension

Humanists recognise that we are products of both our personal and social histories. The fact that our sense of identity is strongly bound up with our relationships and social roles, alerts us to the point that we may have several/**multiple identities**. We 'change' (or at least show different sides of us) in different contexts and at different times in our life.

The humanistic treatment approach

Humanistic therapists apply the humanistic perspective in different ways, but they all agree about the importance of five basic elements.

1. The primary aim of therapy is growth of a positive self-concept.
2. Each person requires *holistic* and individualised treatment.
3. The treatment process should enable a person's special potential, creativity and independence to flourish.

4. Therapists should aim to be warm, genuine, valuing, accepting and non-directive in order to inspire self-acceptance and encourage autonomy.
5. Treatment aims to be client-centred and allow the person to set his or her own agenda.

The main treatment methods/techniques employed are: **subjective accounts** (e.g. encouraging the patient/client to write a diary), **non-directive counselling** (individual or group) and **creative activities** to help individuals gain insight into their feelings and develop greater self-awareness.

THEORY INTO PRACTICE

Basic principles to guide a non-directive therapist

Carl Rogers (1951) developed the non-directive counselling technique which has been applied widely in counselling, and encounter/psychotherapy groups. The technique is used to enable patients/clients to feel comfortable and safe enough to say what they really think/feel. The therapist aims to accept the patient/client – 'warts and all'. The therapist maintains a deep respect for the patient's/client's ability to solve their own situation, and so does not attempt to direct the action/conversation. An over-controlling therapist is giving a message that he or she can control events better than the patient/client.

Virginia Axline has applied these principles to her work doing playtherapy with children. She writes that non-directive counselling or psychotherapy is 'one means of freeing the individual so that he can become a more spontaneous, creative, and happy individual ...' (1989, p. 26). She goes on to say the non-directive therapist is client-centred because 'to him, the client is the source of living power that directs the growth from within himself ...' (1989, p. 22).

Humanistic approach applied to occupational therapy

There are three main ways in which occupational therapy and humanism converge: (a) in our philosophy (b) in our view of the centrality of relationships and (c) in our use of creative activities.

Yerxa has written widely about what she sees as the essentially **humanistic values** underpinning occupational therapy, i.e. optimism, holism and approach to seeing the patient/client as active, autonomous and with a right to life satisfaction (Yerxa, 1983) '... by increasing the client's capacity to be independent we help him perceive himself as possessing worth. He is not a 'thing' to be manipulated helplessly by others but is a human being who can exercise some control over his environment ...' (1967, p. 3).

In common with many psychodynamic therapists, humanistic therapists place much emphasis on establishing an empowering, *therapeutic relationship*. Relationships are seen as crucial to develop a person's self-esteem as well as fulfilling needs. The therapists believe a non-judgmental approach allows a person to express, and thus examine, his or her less desirable feelings or behaviour without fearing censure. Also having another person accept/value you, helps you do the same for yourself.

Finally, humanistic therapists exploit the *potential of creative (and any other) activities*. Creative, spontaneous expression is encouraged. Activities are also valued for helping people be active and productive (and thereby engendering feelings of a sense of achievement and worth). When therapists prescribe activities (any activity from baking to typing to art) – we do so in order to enable individuals to reach their potential, excite their creativity and improve their self-esteem – all humanistic concerns.

THEORY INTO PRACTICE

Applying humanistic concepts in occupational therapy

Consider the following treatment example of how the creative activity of jewellery making helped Teresa to regain her self-esteem.

For 17 years, Teresa, aged 35, was a housewife and mother. Her two children have now left home and her husband has left her for a younger woman. She is depressed and feels she has nothing to offer anyone, let alone herself.

On assessment the therapist felt that: (a) Teresa had spent her life giving to others and now needed to learn to give to herself; and (b) Teresa's low self-esteem was related to her multiple losses and lack of productive activity. In all, Teresa was not doing anything in her life to make her feel good about herself and her abilities.

Jewellery making was an activity which the therapist felt had much therapeutic potential. Teresa had expressed an interest in it, but felt the skill was beyond her. She agreed however to meet weekly with the therapist for a one-to-one jewellery making session where Teresa could talk and work as the mood took her. Initially they started at a relatively 'easy' level, threading small colourful beads. She was pleased with the results and others showed their appreciation when she gave the necklaces as presents. The therapist then encouraged her to make a few pieces for herself as part of valuing herself. Teresa gradually learned new, more difficult skills including enamelling. She really enjoyed creating new designs. Much to her surprise, she found she had an aptitude for jewellery making and she was even able to sell a few pieces. At last she felt she could achieve something beyond being a failed housewife and mother.

The social perspective

'How would you describe yourself?' – I asked four people this question and here is what they said:

Male, white, 50, cross between a builder and an academic, I like travel, sport, scenery, people.

Outgoing, young, lively, I like being with people, I'm interested in them.

… Jewish wife and mother …

I'm a boy, 8 years old, I go to school, I have a dog called Buster.

Notice how most of these descriptions involve references to our social persona and social categories, i.e. our sex/gender, age, class, race/ethnicity/religion, occupations? These form the core elements of our identity. Whilst each individual is unique, we are all linked to others in terms of our **shared social experience**. The social perspective focuses on just this point. It is not really a theory, but an amalgam of theories (e.g. symbolic interactionism and social constructionism) derived from fields of social psychology and sociology. In order to give you a flavour of this vast field of literature I will briefly consider the significance of three different aspects: social roles, social relationships and culture.

Key concepts

Social roles
Roles can be formal/official (e.g. mother, occupational therapist) or informal (e.g. group roles like 'the swot', 'the attention seeker', 'the challenger'). Whatever role we take on they influence how we behave and what we do and say. In social situations, we adopt certain attitudes and behaviours according to our own and other's expectations about how we should behave. These expectations are commonly tied up with perceptions about roles.

One influential social psychology experiment which demonstrates the power of roles was carried out by Zimbardo and his colleagues. They investigated the behaviour of 'ordinary' people which dramatically altered once they were placed into roles of prisoners and guards in a simulated prison. Zimbardo concludes that, '... the mere act of assigning labels to people ... is sufficient to elicit pathological behaviour ...'. He goes on to make a point about contemporary prisons, 'The prison situation ... is guaranteed to generate severe enough pathological reactions in both guards and prisoners as to debase their humanity, lower feelings of self-worth and make it difficult for them to be part of society outside of their prison' (Zimbardo, 1990, p. 176). Here, Zimbardo makes a point about the impact of wider institutions – a point that becomes particularly relevant if we relate it to our patients who are in a *'sick role'*. They are fundamentally affected by the behaviour and attitudes of professionals and the hospital environment.

So what of our other roles – for instance, our work role, a role that has particular significance in occupational therapy? Warr (1987) has extensively researched the psychological effects of the **work role**. He proposes the *'vitamins model'* where, just as we need vitamins for physical health, we need particular elements in our work environment for our mental health. These are: opportunity for control, opportunity for skill use, externally generated goals, variety, availability of money, physical security, opportunity for interpersonal contact and valued social position. Warr considers that different work/jobs can provide sufficient, deficient or toxic levels of these environmental vitamins. Many studies have shown, for example, that giving people more (but not too much) responsibility and control in their work helps to increase their sense of well-being. Research also demonstrates the negative psychological consequences of unemployment, namely, anxiety, depression and low self-esteem. People who are unemployed have less feelings of competence, confidence, sense of control and lower aspirations. Further, they are often in a poverty trap which in itself creates greater anxiety/stress. All these feelings are compounded with detrimental effects on the family. Research like this powerfully demonstrates the importance of our social environment and the social relationships which exist within it.

Social relationships

Our family, friends, colleagues and teachers all clearly have a role in shaping our identity and behaviour. The theories of **symbolic interactionism** and **social constructionism** go one step further and propose that the development of self-identity can only occur through interactions with others. Mead, an influential proponent of this view, asserts, 'Selves can only exist in definite relationships with other selves' (Mead, 1934, p. 1664). This means that if a baby were abandoned on a desert island and miraculously lived to adulthood in the absence of humans, the person would not have any sense of 'self'. Our awareness arises out of our special human capacities of being able to: use language/symbols, be reflexive and be empathetic to the perspectives of others.

Mead considers **socialisation** is a continuing process where self-identity is developed and modified. Primary socialisation occurs in early childhood and centres around the family and significant others. Secondary socialisation starts through school years and continues throughout life. The feedback offered by the people within our work, social and home environment helps us establish our self-definitions, and then enables us to grow and change. The attitudes of people around us are a source of evidence and information about oneself, and they play their part in shaping our attitudes, beliefs and cultural norms.

Culture

The influence of culture is both pervasive and subtle. Much of how we behave and what we believe in is a product of our particular community background. We take our cultural heritage for granted and often do not see that what we consider as 'normal' is in fact **socially constructed**.

One example of the power of culture is how different societies have different concepts of health and illness. 'Wind illness' is one of the most common complaints in societies of Southeast Asia and is a good illustration of this. The condition refers to combinations of physical and mental disorder, plus spiritual possession. A nice account of this illness (and the gap between Western and Eastern medicine) is offered by Eisenbruch (1983). He describes treating a 46-year-old Vietnamese mother living in Britain with a history of chronic headaches, insomnia, anorexia, low motivation, etc. Western diagnosis of depression contrasted with the patient's Eastern view, which ascribed her condition to non-observance of the Chinese post-partum ritual. Not surprisingly, Western medicine proved useless and acupuncture beneficial.

The social perspective applied to therapy

There is no specific method of applying the social perspective as it is relevant in every treatment context – it permeates all aspects of therapy from people to problems.

First, all the treatment approaches discussed earlier recognise social aspects. The psychodynamic approach concentrates on the importance of relationships – both in creating and working through them. Behaviourally orientated treatment can take place in groups and utilise social processes of peer modelling and feedback. Humanistic therapies are grounded in a social perspective as group members explore their identity through the eyes of others.

Secondly, therapists work together in teams within **social institutions**. They and their patients/clients are assigned roles which carry with them certain expectations regarding 'appropriate' behaviour and attitudes. Much of what we aim for in occupational therapy relates to our notions of teaching what we believe are appropriate behaviours and skills given **society's norms**.

Lastly, proponents of the social perspective would argue that the problems and disorders manifested by patients/clients are often *socially constructed*. There are two separate strands to this complex argument. (a) The disorders are often created by **social conditions**, for instance, there is clear evidence to show that poverty, family stress and unemployment are linked with many physical and mental illnesses. (b) Disorders are only problems because they are defined that way by society. Different societies (other cultures or periods of history) will have their own ideas about what is normal/abnormal or healthy/ill. Different **social definitions** and values underpin these ideas and can have powerful consequences.

THEORY INTO PRACTICE

Changing definitions and impact on treatment

An example of how the way we define disorders is culturally specific and how that fundamentally affects treatment is how people with learning disabilities have been 'labelled' over this last century. They have been called imbeciles, cretins, moral defectives, mentally handicapped and now people with learning difficulties or disabilities. The imbeciles and cretins were kept in sub-standard, even sub-human, conditions as 'they didn't know any better'. The moral defectives were locked away to protect society. The handicapped were cared for in special institutions. Now, people with learning disabilities are seen as having full rights to live 'normal' lives and are just in need of extra or special education.

The social perspective applied to occupational therapy

Occupational therapy has its origins in a social perspective. Our very concern with how people function in their daily **life roles** and in their different **social environments** (work, home, community) is fundamentally tied to a social, as opposed to medical, outlook. More specifically, when we plan treatment we take into account an individual's **socio-cultural circumstances**. Also, all our treatments are socially based in that they involve **social relationships** and interaction (either with us or in a group situation).

The following two examples of groupwork demonstrate how a focus of social concepts are relevant in occupational therapy.

Groupwork example 1

Seven patients who are moving towards discharge into the community meet once a week for a 'leisure group'. The group members all have long standing mental health problems and particular difficulties in social interaction. They also tend to be socially isolated when living in the community with very little outlet for leisure pursuits. The weekly leisure group gives these patients a safe, structured opportunity to interact. Each week they go on an outing in the community, e.g. to the local sports centre. These outings are beneficial as the group members can learn how to use local facilities, whilst enjoying themselves.

Groupwork example 2

Six men have come together for a 12 session closed group for men only, held in the community. Using a range of activities such as discussion and role play, these men explore the pressures of what it is like to be a man. They share their difficulties about coping with their mental health problems, unemployment, tensions about how to form appropriate relationships with women and how to get on with other men, etc.

3.2 TWO CASE ILLUSTRATIONS

So far in this chapter we have seen how our view of patients/clients' problems and thus their treatment depends on which theoretical approach we adopt. As described in Chapter 2, theories act rather like different spectacles through which we view the world. The idea that occupational therapists choose treatment based on theory, rather than on objective analysis of the patient's/clients' problems is a confusing one. Analysis is usually underpinned by the therapist's perspective, even if it is implicit rather than explicit. Thus 'objective analysis' is a problematic concept. The fact that problems are understood in different ways, and there is never a 'right' treatment (though there are wrong ones!), can feel frustrating. To help you begin to feel more comfortable with the complexities of contrasting theoretical approaches, I offer two more illustrative case studies where therapists from the four approaches each tell their story.

Case illustration 3.1: 'Katie'

Katie, aged 20, has bulimia nervosa (an eating disorder involving regular binges on huge quantities of food followed by overwhelming guilt and a compulsion to get rid of it by vomiting or purging). She is attractive, slim, intelligent and studying medicine successfully at university. On the face of it she seems to have a lot going for her but underneath the surface she is deeply unhappy and is carrying the dark secret of her condition.

In common with many of her friends, she is concerned to be slimmer and is invariably 'on a diet'. She believes that once she can control her food intake and diet successfully, she will 'become slim and happy'. Currently she is in a vicious cycle of crash dieting half the week, then intensively bingeing and vomiting the other half. Usually her binges are associated with times of high emotion and stress, for instance when she has had an argument with her parents and feels unable to assert her needs.

Katie's course is very stressful and she feels pressured by her parents high expectations of her. She describes always feeling 'a failure' and that she is 'some-how never good enough' for her parents. She has always had a tense relationship (anger is never directly expressed) with both her parents. She perceives her father as critical and abusive and her mother as distant. As a young girl Katie often took responsibility to care for younger brothers as her parents were involved with their careers/social life.

Here is what a **psychodynamic therapist** might say ...

Katie's problems stem from her unhappy and angry relationship with her parents. We can make a number of possible interpretations of what may be happening for her. (a) Its possible for example that her craving for food is symbolic of her needing love. When she binges she is filling a need – com-bating her emptiness. (b) Katie appears to have a deep-seated anger against her parents. She probably resents their critical coldness and how they forced her to grow up too fast in order to parent her younger siblings. She is unable to express that anger, however, as it feels too dangerous and destructive. So she represses it. By pushing food into her mouth, she symbolically pushes her feelings down. Bingeing then becomes a way to stop herself feeling her emotions. (c) Alternatively, the anger she cannot express outwards is turned inwards as she abuses and damages herself.

My recommended treatment would be psychotherapy and/or projective activities to help her uncover and explore her angry, needy feelings related to her parents. Once she has the insight linking issues of control, unex-pressed anger and her eating needs, she will be able to take control of her behaviour.

Here is what a **behavioural therapist** might say..

Katie's main problem is the bingeing–vomiting behaviour. This vicious cycle is aggravated by her distorted attitudes to weight, diet and dieting. It is important to consider the antecedents of her bingeing, i.e. what sets it off? Are there any particular associations/stimuli which are relevant? It seems that she is in the habit of handling her stress by bingeing. What then are the pay-offs to her behaviour? She would not continue with such destructive behaviour unless it was rewarding at some level. The fact that the bingeing is likely to have a tranquillising effect and will be effective at distracting her from other worries must be considered a potential reward. Also, her weight control is clearly a big factor in her vomiting. Her fears of gaining weight becomes a possible negative reinforcer when combined with her distorted understanding of diet.

My recommended treatment would be a three-pronged strategy. (a) Help Katie to examine and modify her attitudes towards food, dieting, her body, i.e. help her see she is not fat and that she will not gain weight if she sticks to three well balanced daily meals. (b) Encourage her to recognise antecedents and pay-offs of her out of control behaviour. (c) Re-train new dietary habits through using a diary. Katie should record all eating related behaviours and these will be discussed weekly with her therapist. This should prove effective as the therapist can positively reinforce (praise) any reduction in bulimic behaviour and Katie will want to avoid publicly failing (negative reinforcement).

Here is what a **humanistic therapist** might say ...

Katie has two main problems: (a) a poor self-concept and (b) unmet emotional needs. In terms of her poor and distorted self-concept, she has an extremely low self-esteem (e.g. always feels a failure) and a negative body image. Her unmet needs concern her feeling of unhappiness. Her eating behaviour is a way of giving to herself to replace the esteem and love needs which aren't being met by others. The fact that her behaviour is so self-abusive relates to her negative self-image. She has perhaps been told she is bad and unworthy so is fulfilling what she sees as others' expectations of her.

My recommended treatment starts first with discovering what Katie would like to work on and do. Treatment is likely to focus on her recognising her successes; gaining support from others and developing self-awareness. We would discuss the idea that she needs to value herself and what she does. In order to feel better about herself, she needs to explore her potential and recognise her successes. Treatment would give her opportunities to succeed and to gain positive feedback from others. Some kind of success experience with a creative activity of her choice, that she values, might be helpful here; otherwise we could focus in on her successes at medical school. Ideally Katie should be given opportunities for one-to-one or group counselling where she can experience support and sharing with others and receive their positive regard. Such groupwork would also be useful to facilitate self-awareness and encourage her self-expression.

Here is what a therapist using a **social perspective** might say ...

Katie's problem needs to be seen as a society-wide, not individual, problem. It is not a coincidence that bulimia nervosa tends to occur in women, given the impossible ideological pressures they face from media images exhorting them to be slim and attractive or feel a failure. It is significant that as media images moved from the thin 'Twiggy' ideals of the 60s towards the more health conscious aerobic jogging culture, the incidence of anorexia decreased and bulimia (where the woman has a more normal weight) has increased. Moreover, we cannot forget that our Western, capitalist, consumer culture has a heavy emphasis (and investment in) on marketing both junk and diet foods.

Because I see Katie's problem is mostly related to a problem with society, my recommended treatment would be at the level of raising social consciousness in women. I would encourage women to 'come out' about their secret and then work together to challenge the pressures of these pernicious feminine ideals. Further, I would encourage women to resist being treated in a medical-model way (e.g. with medication) as this just reinforces sick and passive role behaviours. On a more individual level, I would recommend that Katie join a supportive women's group. Within this group, she can share her experiences and explore any tensions about sexuality, gender roles and expectations.

Case illustration 3.2: 'Peter'

Peter, aged 30, has been in hospital over a period of 2 months suffering with a severe schizophrenic illness. He presents as extremely withdrawn, regressed and confused. His behaviour is bizarre, as he often spends time curled on the floor or rocking stiffly in a chair mumbling to himself. At these times he can become physically aggressive if attempts are made to move him. Peter seems to lack awareness of himself, as evidenced by his behaviour and unkempt appearance. Currently, on the ward, the nurses have to do much for his basic care, and during his withdrawn phases they even have to feed him. During his admission, sporadic attempts have been made to get him involved in occupational therapy, often without success, and prompting verbal abuse, though on occasions he will wander into the occupational therapy department and sit passively in a corner. The team have decided to make a concerted attempt to engage Peter in an active rehabilitation programme, and it has been suggested that the occupational therapist become the 'key worker'.

Four therapists of different theoretical persuasions tell their own story about how to treat Peter using the medium of pottery, they mobilise very different approaches and aims, and these ultimately are shaped by, and depend on, their different theoretical commitments.

The **psychodynamic** approach ...

The occupational therapist's assessment highlighted Peter's (a) aggression – possibly a lot of underlying anger, (b) regression and dependence – indicating his current needs and (c) limited communication – signalling his need for another channel. Her priority in treatment was to develop a nurturing relationship, where Peter could feel safe to engage in activity and begin to express himself.

1. The first stage of treatment was a daily visit to the ward to make contact with Peter – she gently spoke to him without asking for a reply.
2. One day she brought with her a piece of clay, and whilst talking, she made a small figure, and asked if Peter would like it – he nodded.
3. Subsequently, the therapist met with him regularly, talking and playing with the clay, either on the ward or in the department when he showed up.
4. He soon became involved with the claywork, gradually using bigger pieces.

Earlier, the occupational therapist had chosen claywork as it offered a means to make contact and for Peter to regress (with the messiness of the material). Now it was being used projectively, as a way of expressing feelings and channelling aggression (e.g. wedging the clay) – being destructive in a controlled way. Later, treatment would be geared to maintaining the therapeutic relationship and exploring other areas.

The **behavioural** approach …

After assessing Peter, the therapist highlighted three problem areas: (a) self-care, (b) passive behaviour and (c) lack of social interaction. It was decided that the nurses should focus on self-care, whilst the occupational therapist would attempt to 'activate' Peter and engage him in some constructive task behaviour. Discussions revealed that a cup of coffee would be an excellent reinforcer, as Peter loved this drink but was rarely able to have it on the ward.

1. Initially, Peter received a cup of coffee for coming down to the occupational therapy department and staying for half an hour, which proved a highly successful invitation. At these times the therapist stayed with him for increasing periods whilst playing with a piece of clay. When Peter began to show an interest by also playing with the clay, she praised him.
2. On the next day, when he made something, she suggested he have his cup of coffee even though it was earlier than usual. Subsequently he only received coffee when he had used the clay for a period.
3. Increasingly, Peter spent more time with the pottery on his own volition. After a few weeks, and occasional instruction, he produced some attractive pots, and as he earned a good reputation he began to actively seek instruction and increase his skill. Treatment focused on improving his task performance skills.
4. This led to the next phase of treatment, which was to encourage active and appropriate social behaviour.

The **humanistic** approach …

The occupational therapist's assessment highlighted a two-fold concern for Peter, i.e. a lack of self-identity, as associated with his illness and as a result of being in an institution, and lack of any creative self-expression. On the positive side she felt his occasional unsolicited attendance at the department indicated his possible interest, and an attempt to make contact. On reviewing his social background she discovered Peter's past hobby of pottery and clay sculpture.

1. On the next few occasions Peter arrived in the department, the occupational therapist spent a few minutes sitting with him without making demands. She said his name and made comments about the environment. She also indicated her impression that he might be interested in joining some time in the future.
2. One morning, whilst maintaining her consistent approach of gently talking to him, the occupational therapist fiddled with a piece of clay. Increasingly, Peter joined in manipulating the clay. No attempt was made to ask him to 'make something' they just worked side by side.
3. Whilst he remained quiet verbally, in action he tentatively played and interacted with the therapist, through the clay.
4. As their relationship developed, Peter began to talk and be more independently involved with the pottery. The next stage would be to involve him in other creative activities with some wider group/social input.

From the **social perspective ...**

The occupational therapist coming from a social perspective assessed Peter's problems in the following way:

1. Peter's mental health problems may well be a result of difficult relationships at home or have been aggravated by social isolation.
2. He has been unemployed for a number of years and he has had few productive role opportunities – both of these problems will have contributed to his mental health problems.
3. His problems (e.g. withdrawal, passivity, poor self-care) result, in part, from the social consequences of his illness, i.e. being hospitalised for such a long period, detached from any normal roles/routines and social interactions.

The therapist's priority for treatment was to engage him in satisfying, productive role behaviour, and then to begin the process of rehabilitation and resettlement back into the community fairly quickly. Special care would be necessary to ensure long-term, follow-up support.

1. Peter was actively encouraged to come down to the occupational therapy department and work on a one to one basis with the therapist.
2. The therapist made sure she interacted naturally with him and offered him choices and responsibilities where possible. On being offered a choice of activities, he selected pottery.
3. After learning how to make a simple mould pot, Peter was encouraged to teach another new patient the technique.
4. Once a consistent routine of doing pottery was established, the treatment plan was enlarged to include other activities (including doing practical activities in a group context).
5. Peter continued to enjoy his pottery sessions and became reasonably skilled at the basic techniques. On his discharge he was referred to a day centre that had a well established pottery class to enable him to pursue his interest.

3.3 DISCUSSION AND EVALUATION

Comparing the theories

So far in reviewing the perspectives we have concentrated on their differences. However, have you also noticed certain similarities and how they overlap? One instance is how the humanistic and social perspectives converge in their beliefs that self-identity arises, at least in part, from others' perceptions. Also, the humanistic perspective allows for the development of multiple selves given different social contexts. In a different way, the humanistic and psychoanalytic perspectives overlap in their concern for individuals' feelings, needs and motivation. Equally, we can see how the social and behavioural perspectives recognise how behaviour can be influenced by modelling on and imitating others in a peer group. Did you spot these links?

Often perspectives converge in their critique of the other perspectives. It is at this point that we get to the heart of the many theoretical debates that get psychologists going! Here are a couple of well travelled arguments.

First, consider the often quoted **nature versus nurture** debate. Here, we can see the behavioural, humanistic and social perspectives join forces under the nurture banner. They all believe we are subject to various life experiences which 'make' us into who we are. This is in contrast to biologically based theories which assert we are 'born' that way – its our nature, in our genes. Out of the four theories you've been introduced to in this chapter, only the psychodynamic perspective specifically acknowledges the role of biological instincts.

The contrasting concepts of **free-will versus determinism** taps another debate. Humanists avowedly support the view that humans are autonomous and have the capacity to be self-directed, i.e. have free-will. In contrast, the behavioural perspective considers us to be at the mercy of our reinforcement history and cognitive capacities. The social perspective also adopts a relatively determinist stance that we are ultimately constrained by our social and cultural heritage. The psychoanalytic perspective sees people as being driven (determined) by forces (i.e. their unconscious and biology) beyond their control, though accepts a person can actively work to recreate themselves through therapy.

Evaluation

I am often asked when teaching these theoretical approaches, 'Which is the best?'. Unfortunately the answer is not that simple! All the theories have their own strengths and weaknesses. The answer to this question will depend in part on the criteria you bring to bear. They solve different problems in different ways.

The **psychodynamic approach** is based on a rich, comprehensive theory which encompasses biological, psychological and social aspects of development. Erikson redresses criticisms against Freud being too focused on sex and the early years, by offering a more social account of the whole life cycle. Psychodynamic treatments offer much scope for exploring inner feelings/the unconscious. The dynamics underlying mental illness (e.g. traumatic childhood experience and relationships) are well described. Its abstract, unproven assumptions making the validity of psychodynamic ideas difficult to establish remains the weakness of this perspective. Also, much of the theory and practice is based on subjective interpretations. Critics say these often reveal more about the psychoanalyst than the patients!

The **cognitive-behavioural perspective**, in contrast, offers a more objective account of human behaviour and relies on proven, systematic methods of scientific research. Behavioural methods of treatment are effective and produce tangible results such as clear behavioural change. However, the methods can be seen as superficial as they do not tackle the underlying cause of a problem behaviour – thus, the problem behaviour will often re-emerge. For instance, an unhappy/angry child may continue to be naughty (though perhaps in a different way) if one behaviour is stopped. Behaviourism is inclined to be mechanistic, rigid and focused narrowly on small elements of behaviour to the detriment of the whole person. You can teach a child a new skill, but what of his/her thoughts, feelings, motivations, to say nothing of wider social aspects? Whilst cognitive and social processes have recently been attended to, the approach is still criticised for insufficiently recognising a person's whole experience.

The **humanistic perspective** takes the idea of the 'whole' person very much on board and recognises wider aspects of human nature – our needs and potential. Humanism allows for our active, reflective capacity and how we can consciously choose a course of action, i.e. we are not simply at the mercy of internal or external drives. However, all the other perspectives would hotly debate the notion that humans are completely free agents. The humanistic perspective remains vague/'waffley'. Its therapy methods (e.g. unconditional positive regard) can be unrealistic and insufficiently focused.

It is hard to disagree with the comprehensive account of social forces offered by **the social perspective**. All the perspectives recognise (to differing degrees) the power of social relationships and culture. Unlike the other perspectives however, the social perspective cannot explain why individuals in the same social and family environment behave so differently. Whilst the social perspective can identify wider social processes at work (e.g. racial and gender divisions in society), their precise effects and their influence on individuals cannot be predicted. Furthermore, this perspective is limited in that it does not offer us any specific therapeutic tools or techniques. It remains a rather general analysis.

Deciding which theory to use

Having established each theory has strengths and weaknesses, how do we know which to use in our clinical practice with patients/clients? Our choice is guided by many factors including: the methods in vogue at the time; the theoretical bias of our team/unit; practical constraints such as time/resources; and our own leanings taking into account our preferences and skills.

Ultimately, we must choose a theoretical framework to suit our particular patient/client – one he or she will accept and one which suits their problem area. Where a problem looks to be a reasonably straightforward behaviour or skill problem (e.g. managing anxiety or learning how to cook), then a cognitive-behavioural approach may be best. Where a problem appears to be more long standing and resists easy solutions, then a longer term more psychodynamically or socially orientated programme might be more effective. Where the problem seems related to low self-esteem, lack of confidence and confused feelings generally, then the humanistic approach comes into its own. In practice, we select which approach appears to be most useful and effective given the particular situation, the person, their problems and needs.

CONCLUSION

During the course of this chapter we have explored why we employ psychological approaches and some of the theories that are available for our use. The key concepts and practical applications of four psychological approaches – psychodynamic, cognitive-behavioural, humanistic and social – were discussed and illustrated (see summary in Table 3.1). I hope I have shown the profound and subtle influence of theory on how we 'understand' patients' problems, and how we apply treatment. Basically each theory aids therapists in two main ways: it functions as an *analytical tool* to help us understand our patient's/client's problems more fully and it suggests a particular *treatment method*.

Table 3.1 Summary of the four psychological approaches and their application

Theory	Key concepts	Focus of assessment	Treatment activities
Psychodynamic	developmental stages, dynamic unconscious	unconscious needs, relationships, ego organisation	psychotherapy, creative and projective activities
Cognitive-behavioural	learning and conditioning, cognition	task performance, skills, behaviour	behaviour therapy, skills training, practical activities
Humanistic	self-concept, autonomy, freedom, needs/feelings	self concept, needs, situation	creative therapies and any valued activity
Social	social categories, roles, relationships, culture	social situation and needs, social impact and meanings of disorder	group work, family therapy, community and leisure groups

I have also tried to demonstrate how each approach has specific strengths and offers useful insight into some aspects of human development. Each has weaknesses in terms of its assumptions and the way it omits certain factors in its analysis.

Our awareness of competing perspectives acts as a healthy challenge and critique of our own views and practices. Whatever choice of perspective we make as therapists, it needs to be an informed one. We have a professional responsibility to understand the logic, strengths, weaknesses, similarities and contrast among the different theories in order to apply them effectively. This knowledge and understanding is essential to enable us to communicate with other members of the team and to implement a coherent treatment programme.

Discussion questions

1. How do we chose what theoretical approach to apply in treatment?
2. Does our use of directive and behavioural techniques contradict our essentially humanistic values?
3. Occupational therapists should not use psychodynamic techniques without further training. Discuss.
4. Consider one of the case illustrations offered in Chapter 2. To what extent would the treatment have differed had psychological approaches been used?
5. It is better to maintain a commitment to one theoretical approach rather than taking an eclectic stance. Discuss.
6. To what extent are occupational therapists who use psychological approaches encroaching on other professionals' territory?

<table>
<tr><td>**4**</td><td># Assessment</td></tr>
</table>

Assessment is the first stage of the occupational therapy process, and consists of gathering information in an effort to understand the patient/client and his/her situation. In terms of a problem-solving process, assessment aims to understand the problem and how it affects the person or persons involved. It is of vital importance as treatment can only be effective if the assessment accurately identifies the person's problem and situation.

This chapter aims to explore different aspects of the assessment process. First, the assessment process is put into a context by answering the questions of why? what? when? and how? Secondly, different methods of assessment are analysed and their use evaluated. Particular attention will be paid to the range of published (though not necessarily standardised) tools. Lastly, I will discuss a range of practical and ethical questions about assessment, recognising the wider implications of it in practice.

4.1 WHY? WHAT? WHEN? HOW?

Why do we assess?

Careful, accurate assessment is vital if effective treatment is to be applied. After all, how can we know what to treat, and to what level, if we have not specifically identified the area of need? Further, how can we treat people as individuals if we have not discovered what is special about them?

As a problem solver, the occupational therapist needs to be clear about the problem and its parameters. Consider the therapist who is referred a patient who 'lacks concentration'. In order to plan treatment, he or she needs to find out:

1. What exactly is meant by this? What happens (e.g. lapses into non-productive behaviour)? When does this occur (e.g. during tasks)? How does this affect the individual's functioning (e.g. unable to return to the task)? Here the problem is specifically defined.

2. How many minutes can the individual concentrate when carrying out daily tasks? This becomes the baseline to measure any improvement.
3. What situations increase/decrease concentration? This is important both to help the patient/client to develop strategies to cope better with the problem and to enable the occupational therapist to plan a graded treatment.
4. What level of concentration ability does the patient require for daily living? For example, a university student about to take exams and a long-stay patient likely to remain in hospital require qualitatively different levels of concentration. This information is needed to establish the aim of treatment.

If these questions are not answered the resulting treatment stands in danger of being stereotyped (i.e. not recognising the individual's needs), 'waffley' (i.e. lacking specific goals) and possibly completely ineffective (e.g. may end up working on the wrong problem!).

The process of assessment continues throughout treatment. Having established the baseline problem/issues, progress can be evaluated by reassessing the person's functioning and comparing the current and previous results.

Thus, assessment is important in order to: (a) understand the problem/s, (b) recognise the person's individual needs, (c) identify the baseline for treatment and (d) evaluate progress.

What do we assess?

Assessment is the first stage of the occupational therapy process. It involves the gathering of information, from any relevant source, about the person and his or her circumstances. Our assessments will normally focus on how individuals cope with their daily life *occupations* in work, leisure and self-care. Specifically, the assessment should pinpoint a person's *functional skills and problems* related to emotional, cognitive, social and physical areas. But in order to understand this, the assessment needs to probe something about *the individual*: his or her needs, interests, motivations and strengths. These are the positive areas on which treatment is built. The assessment also needs to take into account the person's *social situation* including expected environment (including the amount of support available) and cultural practices or meanings, as these will determine long-term treatment aims (see Figure 4.1).

Our general focus on occupational performance needs to be seen within the context of the assessments made by other team members. Importantly each team member should have a slightly different focus according to their role and concerns. Not only would it be a waste of time and effort (everybody's) simply to duplicate each others assessments, it is impossible for one member to cover all areas at once. Ideally the team should have an overall strategy for assessment where a division of labour is negotiated which ensures different areas of a patient's/client's life are covered by different team members. At the same time there should be some overlap. Often in hospitals for example, doctors and nurses take primary responsibility for assessing patients' mental state during the acute stages of their treatment, whilst the social workers and occupational therapists become involved at the later stages assessing the person's needs and functioning as related to discharge. In this way although the assessments carried out by individual team members are partial, the overall assessment strategy is more holistic.

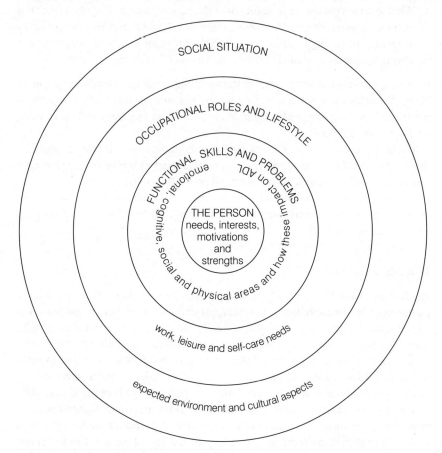

Figure 4.1 Areas for occupational therapy assessment.

When do we assess?

Assessment occurs at all points during treatment – initially, subsequently and continuously (see Figure 4.2). In the initial stages the occupational therapist (and whole treatment team) will be involved in collecting data – observing, interviewing, testing the patient/client (and possibly the family). The information that is collected will then be analysed, preferably in negotiation with the individual, to consider the priority problems and central issues to be dealt with during treatment. Further specific assessments may then occur at set times according to need (e.g. every fortnight

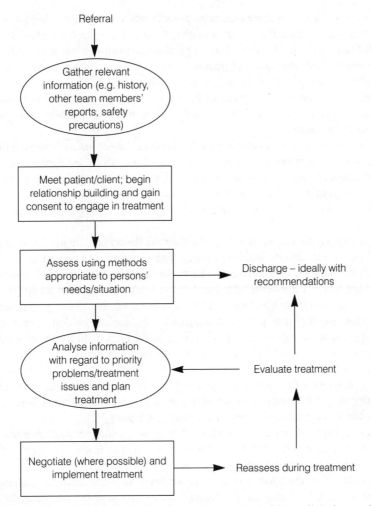

Figure 4.2 The assessment process. Key: box, patient contact; ellipse, clinical reasoning.

or prior to discharge home). At the continuous level, however, assessment is ongoing throughout treatment and the therapist tries to be alert to the patient's/client's responses and any new cues. (One example of such a cue is when a patient mentions he had seen his child that weekend and the therapist, alert to this new information that he is a part-time parent, takes the opportunity to discuss it further.)

How do we assess?

The assessment process (see Figure 4.2) should be seen as part of treatment. Arguably it is the most important part since our treatment is likely to be 'wrong' if we get our assessment 'wrong'.

The initial stages of the assessment process sets the scene for subsequent treatment as this is where the therapist begins to *establish a rapport* and relationship with the patient/client. Sensitively applied assessment can mean the difference between success and failure of treatment. For one thing, the assessment period is the stage where patients/clients give their consent and become engaged in treatment. Further, encouraging patients/clients to be actively involved in their treatment agenda gives them both control and responsibility which will usually increase their motivation.

The next stage of assessment includes the *actual mechanics* of carrying out the assessment. Therapists should try to adopt methods which are appropriate to the patients/clients needs and situation. For example, a patient who is very withdrawn, may well respond better to a non-verbal task than an interview, whilst a patient suffering from performance anxiety and high emotion might prefer initially to talk.

As with any treatment, it is important for the therapist to be *flexible and adapt* the assessment activity when necessary. For example, if a person is becoming overly anxious during a standardised test, the therapist might decide either to suspend the test or offer some additional assistance/support (which would in effect nullify the test). Likewise, we should respond sensitively to our patients/clients when they say they are 'not up to talking today' or 'don't fancy doing occupational therapy'. If we are genuinely handing over some responsibility for treatment to our patients/clients, we have to accept such consequences!

The final stages of the assessment process involves *analysing* and (where possible) *sharing* the findings. Treatment or future interventions can then be planned and negotiated. Of course assessment doesn't end there. We continue to assess and evaluate throughout the person's treatment (see Figure 4.2).

The assessment process is neither a linear, nor a completely systematic procedure. Sometimes the therapist seems to function at an instinctive level and may even be unaware of picking up on an individual's subtle verbal and non-verbal behaviour. The therapist may also make imaginative assessment judgements which seem to be based on 'gut feeling' rather than tangible evidence. In other words the therapist's clinical reasoning is multi-layered.

THEORY INTO PRACTICE

Assessment involves multi-level clinical reasoning

Scientific reasoning
On receiving a referral the therapist is likely to formulate some provisional and tentative ideas. For instance, on being given a diagnosis, the therapist could estimate information about length of treatment, prognosis, level of individual's insight and cognitive function.

Narrative reasoning
Then the therapist sets out on an initial interview to build a relationship with the individual concerned. Together they build a picture of the individual's particular

needs and situation. For example, the patient discloses she is being abused by her husband but fears being alone in the future and having to cope as a single mother.

Interactive reasoning
Throughout the assessment and as the relationship and therapy evolves, the therapists adapt their approach in response to the patient's/client's cues. For example, when a therapist sees his patient is lacking in motivation during an activity, he suggests they take a break in order to work out what is going wrong.

Pragmatic reasoning
As they work together to plan a treatment, the therapist considers wider social factors and practical constraints. For instance, the therapist knows the patient is likely to be discharged within 2 weeks so does not consider in-depth treatment options.

The most important point for therapists to remember is that the assessments are *tools* to be used judiciously and selectively. Some patients/clients will respond well to an informal assessment approach, such as coming to 'have a chat' whilst they make a cup of tea. Others could find this patronising and would not perceive it as a professional approach, preferring instead to have a more formal, structured procedure. Therapists judgement, even intuition, clearly plays a part in deciding what assessment to apply, as well as how and when to apply it. The effective assessor enacts both the science and art of therapy.

4.2 METHODS OF ASSESSMENT

There are many different types of assessment available for our use – some standardised and/or published, some developed and practised locally. Basically we have five formal methods of eliciting information about our patients/clients: (a) standardised tests, (b) interview, (c) structured observation, (d) self-rating and (e) psychodynamic activities. These will be described in turn, considering their aims and type of information they can elicit, alongside issues surrounding their application in practice. Most sections also include information on some useful, well researched, published tools.*

Standardised tests

A standardised test is a formal procedure which has been carefully researched and practised, increasing its objective and 'scientific' status. Three main elements need to be addressed when standardising a test:

* Some published assessments are fully standardised in that they have: (a) established reliability/validity, (b) test norms and (c) detailed administration instructions. Other published tools (e.g. the many published tools from the US arising from the Model of Human Occupation) only fit some of these criteria. For this reason, I prefer to distinguish between 'published' and 'standardised' or at least to view them along a continuum of how well they have been researched.

- The test norm should be defined, i.e. the accepted standard given a particular population needs establishing.
- A consistent clear administrative procedure and scoring system needs to be developed and used by specifically trained assessors.
- The instrument's validity and reliability must be established (i.e. does the test measure what it is supposed to in a consistent way across assessors and time?), with many trials after which adjustments may be made.

Most of the assessments we use in occupational therapy (including many of the published tools) are not standardised. Research (e.g. McAvoy, 1991; Hammond, 1996) indicates therapists lack knowledge of and access to what is available. The fact that we tend to use non-standardised assessments does not negate their value, but should alert us to the importance of approaching any results with caution. With some time and extra research, many of our tests currently in use could achieve the 'standardised' label.

The pool of standardised tests (and different norm tables) available is increasing every year as demand grows for valid assessments and reliable outcome measures. Some of the more widely used assessments in the UK are the 'Clifton', 'Rivermead', 'Adaptive Behaviour Scale', 'FPR', Life Experience Checklist and 'COTNAB'. Recently the AMPS, based on the Model of Human Occupation, has generated much interest around the world as it is a specifically devised occupational therapy test which both measures skill components and functioning in activities of daily living. Each of these are discussed below.

With all standardised tests, four points need to be stressed to avoid their misuse/abuse:

1. It is important that the assessors are *properly trained* to administer and score the test according to standard methods, maximising the test's reliability and validity. The AMPS test, for example, requires the user to attend a 5 day course. For information on other courses available that train therapists in the use of specified standardised tests contact the College of Occupational Therapists, 6–8 Marshalsea Road, London SE1 1HL.
2. Testing is not just a matter of following procedure – it also requires *interpretation of results*. Here the occupational therapist requires a good understanding about the rationale behind the test and the comparisons with available norms. Without this tests remain observational tools only.
3. Each test has *limitations* and weaknesses. Tests are usually designed for specific populations, types of problems and/or situations, and are only applicable to such areas. Some tests are weak in certain areas, such as being vague with their instructions. Also, some tests stir up considerable performance tensions in people, which could unduly affect the result (to say nothing about the patient's/client's response to occupational therapy as a whole).
4. Care must be taken when reporting any results and making *recommendations*. If a test is not administered precisely (for instance if tasks are modified or the client prompted) it may invalidate the assessment. It is legitimate (and may

even be desirable) to adapt an assessment, as long as we do not report results as being produced by a standardised procedure. As de Clive-Lowe (1996) warns, clinicians need to use tests responsibly.

Overall, standardised assessments offer an objective, systematic and scientific way of assessing patients/clients. Whilst they are invaluable for comparing results and demonstrating findings to other professionals, they remain a tool to be used alongside other (perhaps non-standardised) tools.

Published tools

CAPE – The Clifton Assessment Procedures for the Elderly (Pattie and Gilleard, 1979)

This assessment was developed by psychologists to be used by 'all those professionally concerned with the care and management of the elderly'. The procedures involve tests consisting of two scales designed to assess cognitive and behavioural competence. These are:

- The cognitive assessment scale which measures knowledge/orientation (by quiz-type questions), mental ability (by counting, reading, etc.) and psychomotor skill (by tracing a spiral maze).
- The behaviour rating scale which considers physical disability, apathy, communication and social disturbance. Comparison of the results with available norms allows the therapist to assess the degree of dependence present, indicating the levels of care and support needed.

The strength of this assessment is that it involves an easily learned and applied procedure, i.e. the therapist only needs to become familiar with the manual. The resulting clearcut scores determining levels of dependency offer a certain amount of security. The test has been widely used throughout the UK (particularly with the large-scale resettlement of elderly people from long-stay hospitals into the community) by many professional groups which confers a certain amount of legitimacy on it. Arguably it is a less relevant tool for occupational therapists who would normally be more involved with assessing actual ADL functioning and occupational performance rather than using paper and pencil measures.

This package can be obtained from: NFER-Nelson Publishing Co. Ltd, Darville House, 2 Oxford Road East, Windsor, Berkshire SL4 1DF. This firm will supply standardised tests to named individuals qualified to use them and also offers demonstration workshops if needed.

The Rivermead Perceptual Assessment Battery (Whiting et al., 1985)

This assessment is one of the more widely used standardised perceptual tests available for occupational therapists in the UK. It consists of a battery of 16 timed tests (taking approximately 1 hour to administer). Tasks range from matching simple pictures to copying a complex three-dimensional model. The assessment is designed to measure deficits in visual perception and so is most relevant for assessing people with schizophrenia or with neurological disorders.

Its main values are that it has been well produced and researched. It is relatively easy to apply although care needs to be taken to follow the instructions precisely. Some patients/clients find the formality and timed elements stressful, whilst others appreciate its professional presentation. Arguably its focus on visual perception limits its value and broader cognitive-perceptual tests, such as the COTNAB, may be more useful.

The manual contained in the assessment package includes information on interpretation of scores, and illustrative therapy case studies. This battery can be obtained from: NFER-Nelson Publishing Co. Ltd, Darville House, 2 Oxford Road East, Windsor, Berkshire SL4 1DF.

Adaptive Behaviour Scale (Nihara, Leland and Lambert, 1993)

The Adaptive Behaviour Scale – Residential and Community (ABS – RC:2) defines adaptive behaviour as having coping abilities to allow for a 'reasonably normal lifestyle'. It has been designed to be used for people with learning disabilities (norms available) but can be applied to other groups. It is a primarily an observational tool (or carried out in discussion with carers). This scale has been in use in various stages of development since 1969. This current community focused edition consists of two parts: (a) personal independence, which assess areas such as personal ADL, sensory and motor development, money handling and shopping, self-direction, and (b) social behaviour, which takes into account expectations of the public and covers social behaviour, conformity, trustworthiness, etc. Some training is necessary to handle the scoring scale and norm tables.

The ABS is sensitive to degrees of handicap and offers a good overview of skills which acts as a baseline measure for treatment evaluation. It is relatively easy to administer, and although it takes some time to carry out it can be approached more selectively. Studies support the validity of the ABS and it has been used as an outcome measure for research purposes.

The assessment is available from: NFER-Nelson Publishing Co. Ltd, Darville House, 2 Oxford Road East, Windsor, Berkshire SL4 1DF.

FPR – Functional Performance Record

The FPR assesses 26 topic areas including activity levels, aggression, domestic and survival skills, mobility, personal hygiene, and the use of transportation. The items are rated selectively on the basis of actual observed behaviour (by therapist or carer) over the last week. The FPR is a computerized checklist (on disc) where therapists input data and a graph of percentage deficit is produced.

The strength of this assessment is its scientific approach and computerized format. The visual readout offers a clear profile of functioning and is a useful tool for communicating with clients or carers. Whilst the percentage deficit approach goes slightly against our philosophy of emphasising ability and being holistic, it charts minute progress. This is a useful assessment for assessing people who are elderly or who have a range of functional problems in that physical, psychological and social functioning is considered.

The assessment is available from: NFER-Nelson Publishing Co. Ltd, Darville House, 2 Oxford Road East, Windsor, Berkshire SL4 1DF.

Life Experiences Checklist (Ager, 1990)
The Life Experience Checklist is used primarily with people with learning disabilities and identifies whether deficits in clients' cognitive learning is a result of limitations in cognitive skills or lack of opportunities to learn. The interview questions asked touch on areas to do with home, leisure, relationships, freedom and opportunity. The yes/no questions (which can be answered by the client or therapist on the client's behalf) are appropriately straightforward, for instance: 'My home has more rooms than people'; 'My home is carpeted and has comfortable furniture' or 'I visit friends and relatives for a meal once a month'. Scoring with norms is standardised against the general population (recognising urban, suburban and rural differences).

The checklist is quickly administered and can be used flexibly as an individual assessment tool or for group treatment. Although very simple, it offers a useful insight into the person's quality of life and pinpoints possible environmental problems.

The assessment is available from: NFER-Nelson Publishing Co. Ltd, Darville House, 2 Oxford Road East, Windsor, Berkshire SL4 1DF.

COTNAB – The Chessington Occupational Therapy Neurological Assessment Battery
The COTNAB is one of several assessments occupational therapists can use to assess neurological functioning (e.g. who have suffered a head injury or stroke). There are 12 sub-tests which assess: (a) visual perception (overlapping figures, hidden figures and sequencing), (b) constructional ability (two-dimensional, three-dimensional and spatial ability), (c) sensory motor ability (stereognosis, dexterity and hand-eye co-ordination); and (d) ability to follow instructions (written, visual and spoken). The patient's/client's scores on each test are compared with norms for that age group in terms of ability, time and overall performance.

This professionally packaged (but expensive) assessment is one of the best known tools as it was specifically designed for occupational therapists' use. It has a good research base (see, e.g. Sloan *et al.*, 1991; Laver and Hutchinson, 1994). COTNAB is often favoured by therapists over the Rivermead as it tests wider cognitive function as opposed to just visual perception. In common with the Rivermead, the limitations of this test are the performance tensions it can generate. On the other hand, people also enjoy carrying out the interesting and challenging puzzles/tasks.

COTNAB is available from: Nottingham Rehab Ltd, Ludlow Hill Road, West Bridgford, Nottingham NG2 6HD.

AMPS – Assessment of Motor and Process Skills (Fisher, 1994)

The AMPS simultaneously assesses functional performance in ADL tasks (like meal preparation) and underlying motor/cognitive skills. The person carries out a specifically defined ADL task of choice whilst the assessor (who is specifically trained and 'calibrated') carefully observes. Sixteen motor and 20 process skill items are scored using a four-point rating scale (4 = competent, 1 = deficit). The scores are then analysed by computer using the many faceted Rasch analysis to provide measures which are adjusted to account for the challenge of the task, severity of the rater, the ability of the subject and the difficult of the skill items.

The strength of this assessment is its highly scientific approach. First, a number of studies have supported its validity and reliability (see, e.g. Robinson and Fisher, 1996) and its clinical research base is developing (e.g. Baron, 1994). Secondly, the computer scoring of the precise level of motor and process skills allows therapists to predict how well a client can be expected to perform on many other ADL tasks. On the negative side, some therapists feel uncomfortable with using this tool as the requirements to ensure reliability can be restrictive. Tasks need to be done a certain way (or will be scored down) which may not suit individual's own methods. Early problems with cross cultural applications are being attended to as research and training around the world grows (allowing a bigger pool of data).

Assessors need to attend a 5-day training and calibration workshop (held in the UK and around the world) to develop the skills for scoring and interpreting results. Therapists wishing to attend should contact: AMPS Project, Occupational Therapy Building, Colorado State University, Fort Collins, CO 80523, USA.

Interviews

Interviews are the use of structured conversation to gain insight into a person's world. They are most widely used as our initial assessment tool, and often are the only more formal procedure the occupational therapist applies alongside informal, general observations and interactions with the patient/client. As Mosey comments, 'Interviewing is probably the most powerful, sensitive and versatile evaluative instrument available to the occupational therapist' (1986, p. 314).

Aims

Different interviews do different jobs. Thus the interview that takes place as the first contact between therapist and patient/client is primarily a relationship-building exercise, with the occupational therapist sharing as much information about his or her role as the patients/clients share about their situation. Subsequent treatment-planning interviews will have a more specific focus regarding the person's attitudes, interests and view of problems he or she is prepared to work on.

The main aim of the interview is to gain information from the patient/client, considering both what is said and how he or she says it. At a verbal level we seek to tap relevant factual information, like situation and interests, as well as feelings/attitudes and the person's own view of his or her problems. Through listening we can also obtain information regarding verbal skills and intellectual capacities. At a non-verbal level the person's appearance and behaviour may communicate much about their mood, mental state and attitudes. What specific information is obtained depends not only on the individual's specific problems, but also on his or her motivation, abilities and situation.

Application

Any interview must be planned carefully, considering its specific aims and structure, as well as other factors such as the context of the interview and the individual's previous experiences (e.g. of occupational therapy). Prior to the interview the therapist should be clear about what he or she hopes to achieve and why, whilst also being flexible and sensitive to the needs of the situation. Is the interview primarily relationship building? If so, the emphasis should perhaps be on a more informal basis (cups of tea and tours around the occupational therapy department are occasionally helpful here!). Is the interview more a fact-finding mission? Here the therapist can usefully go into the situation armed with a few already formulated, pertinent questions. This pre-empts vague interviews, and can help in those moments when we 'go blank' and do not know what to ask next.

The structure of the interview process itself is, of course, determined by its aims. In general, however, there are two important guidelines:

- Be an *active listener* (more easily said than done), where effort is put into listening instead of formulating your next question.
- Ask *open-ended* questions, such as 'How are you settling in?' as opposed to 'Do you like this ward?' or 'What does your typical day look like?' as opposed to 'Do you have a job?' This way of asking questions allows a person more opportunities to expand his or her comments, and open out, rather than responding with a 'yes' or 'no' answer. Further, it implicitly respects the individual's capacity to take responsibility to share what is important for them. A possible exception to this, however, is when an acutely ill patient seems to need the structure of a simple, direct question.

As a general rule the environment should enable individuals to feel comfortable and safe, in order to encourage them to open up. Often a quiet room off the main ward or a quiet area with which they are familiar is a good start. The key to ensuring 'safety' is to try to respond to what works for each individual. Whilst some people would react positively to a relaxed, informal approach, others may experience this as unprofessional and would prefer a more structured, formal interaction. Safety and trust is also promoted by listening sensitively, giving enough time and being free from interruptions.

Other factors to consider when preparing for an interview include the person's skills and past experiences. One rather thoughtless institutional practice, for example, arises when a patient/client is given a number of interviews by several professionals, all asking similar questions. Consider the not uncommon occurrence of a newly admitted acutely anxious patient, who in the first week may be seen for an initial interview by several doctors and nurses, as well as a range of therapists all with their attached students. We need to strike a balance between checking information from previous reports, showing an interest and gaining useful information. It is important for occupational therapists to decide the particular focus of their questions in view of their particular role (e.g. questions about current problems in functioning would be more relevant than questions about the quality of delusions, on which the medical staff would focus).

THEORY INTO PRACTICE

Five important guidelines for interviewing

The five most important guidelines to bear in mind when interviewing are:

1. Ensure the environment is as 'safe' as possible to encourage the patient/client to feel comfortable and open up.
2. Be an active listener. Put effort into really listening as opposed to formulating the next question (easier said than done!).
3. Ask open-ended questions such as 'What does your typical day entail?' as opposed to 'Do you have a job?'. This gives the person an opportunity to expand on questions whilst allowing him or her to select what is important to share.
4. Respect what it must feel like as the person being interviewed. We are privileged to receive any information, let alone the deep confidences often offered.
5. Remember that assessment is part of the overall treatment. The patient/client needs to understand what it is all about to be motivated to answer. It helps to explain why you need to know the answers to the questions you are asking.

Published tools

OPHI – Occupational Performance History Interview (Kielhofner, Henry and Walens, 1989)
This semi-structured interview was devised as a generic interview tool and is suitable for most occupational therapy contexts (and different theoretical frameworks). Questions are designed to elicit information about a person's past and present occupational routines, life role, interests/values/goals, perception of ability/responsibility and environmental influences. A rating scale offers a way of quantifying information, whilst space is available for a 'life history narrative' to capture qualitative information. This assessment is currently being revised so readers should look out for the up-dated version.

The strength of this assessment is its historical approach in that problems are seen in the context of a person's previous functioning. Given this, it is most useful for assessing people who have been changed (e.g. a person who used to be an alcoholic and now has stopped drinking or someone who had functioned well and then suffered a breakdown or sustained a traumatic injury). The five areas of questioning offer a useful and comprehensive structure without overly constraining the therapist's style of questioning. Less experienced interviewers sometimes prefer a more structured tool. The emphasis on qualitative information and the limited question structure means that inter-rater and test–re-test reliability is reduced. The OPHI works best if the therapist can develop a conversational style. For an in-depth evaluation of the use of this assessment, see Fossey (1996).

The OPHI manual (consisting of instructions, research base information, question lists and scoring forms) can be ordered from: American Occupational Therapy Association Inc., 4720 Montgomery Lane, PO Box 31220, Bethesda, MD 20824-1220, USA.

OCAIRS – Occupational Case Analysis Interview and Rating Scale (Kaplan and Kielhofner, 1989)
This semi-structured interview, arising from the model of human occupation, has been designed for use in the field of acute mental health. Questions are carefully worded to cover all areas of occupational performance, namely, interest, roles, habits, skills, personal causation, values/goals and other areas related to how the individual functions within the environment. The answers are then scored to aid treatment and discharge planning.

The strength of this interview is its clear and comprehensive structure. Therapists new to interviewing often find the supplied set questions helpful. Most (not all) of the questions are written in a user-friendly manner, such as 'How do you like to spend your time'; 'Overall, how satisfied are you with how you spend your time?' and 'What do you see yourself doing 1 year from now?'. More experienced therapists may find the structure too constraining and rigid. The specific and detailed rating scale is both a strength and a weakness in that inter-rater reliability is increased but at the same time it can be hard to rate individuals who do not fit neatly into the headings offered.

The assessment consists of a manual, instructional audio tape and question/rating forms. This package can be purchased from: Slack Inc., 6900 Grove Road, Thorofare, NJ 08086, USA.

WRI – Worker Role Interview (Velozo, Kielhofner and Fisher, 1992)
The WRI is a semi-structured interview and observation tool, based on the model of human occupation. It aims to identify the psycho-social and environmental variables which may influence the ability of the 'injured' worker to return to work. It is designed to enable the client to discuss various aspects of his or her life and job setting that are relevant to past work experience. The recommended questions cover: (a) the effects of injury (e.g. 'What parts of your job do you feel you are unable to do because of your injury?'), (b) life outside of work (e.g. 'What do you do in the evenings'), (c) present job (e.g. 'What are you most proud of in terms of your work?'), (d) past jobs (e.g. 'What other jobs have you had over the last 5 years?') and (e) return to work (e.g. 'Do you think you will return to work?'). The therapist then rates (both interview and work assessment observations) in terms of

content areas based on the model of human occupation (i.e. personal causation, values, interests, roles, habits and environment). Each content area is sub-divided into specific work related issues. For instance, the sub-content area of 'expectation of job success' is rated on a four point scale as to how strongly this item supports the client returning to work. The User's Guide offers detailed instructions for rating individual's responses. Scores obtained on an initial assessment and discharge reassessment may then be compared.

Arguably this assessment has limited value in the psycho-social field given the realities of the employment market. However, it could prove to be a useful tool for any work rehabilitation programme. The strength of this interview is its clear and comprehensive structure. The fact that the interview goes beyond work questions could be seen as both a strength and a limitation (as its extends the interview time). Questions are reasonably user-friendly. The detailed guidelines offered for the scoring system increases the reliability and validity of the assessment. The assessment is still in its early stages of development and the authors would welcome any feedback on the usefulness of the instrument in a clinical setting.

The manual can be obtained from: Model of Human Occupation Clearinghouse, Department of Occupational Therapy M/C 811, University of Illinois at Chicago, 1919 West Taylor Street, Chicago, IL 60657, USA.

Structured observation

Observation is of course the method of assessment we are using all the time. We continuously, often without thinking, monitor (and then respond to) how our patients/clients are presenting, behaving and performing. We try to note how they are reacting to others, their treatment activity and the environment. Structured observation is a more formal systematic procedure where we focus on specific areas (e.g. observing the way a task is being performed or taking note of environmental constraints on a home visit).

The therapists who are particularly skilled at observing, learn to focus on specific and relevant cues. General observations like 'John is looking better today' are transformed into 'John's posture is more upright today, making him look more confident'. It is this level of specific observation which we need to encourage in ourselves for two main reasons. Primarily if we are more specific about a patient's/client's areas of skills or behaviour we then have a more specific baseline for treatment. A second not unimportant factor concerns our professional presentation and our communication with other staff. Our occasionally vague verbal reports can have far-reaching negative consequences.

Application

To help us observe more effectively it may be helpful to utilise one or two of the infinite number of observation checklists available. For instance, many of our *activities of daily living* checklists can be a useful prompt to highlight points such as in the following:

Making a cup of tea   *Comment*
    aware of use of equipment
    organises task in sequence
    aware of safety factors
    fills kettle appropriately
    turns on gas/electricity switches
    puts tea in pot/cup appropriately
    pours boiled water in appropriately
    uses sugar/milk appropriately
    …

Further we can take any developmental chart and translate it into behavioural forms, as the following example detailing the cognitive function at a 2- to 3-year-old level demonstrates. Having such a structure for observations helps us be clear and precise.

                    Date achieved   *Comment*
    draws vertical lines
    copies circle
    matches three colours
    points to big/little in imitation
    places objects 'in' on request
    …

Specific observations like these can be applied to many situations and tasks. They offer an objective measure of performance (though it cannot be called standardised) whereby a patient's/client's actual functioning can be observed rather than inferred.

Published tools

COTE – Comprehensive Occupational Therapy Evaluation (Brayman and Kirby, 1982)
A useful, structured observation scale used primarily for initial assessment is the COTE scale (see Figure 4.3). It has been used widely in the US and is currently applied in the UK under a variety of guises. In addition to the basic scale there are official definitions attached detailing the problems at a specific level to maximise reliability as the following example shows.

    1. Appearance – the following six factors are involved: clean skin, clean hair, hair combed, clean clothes, clothes ironed and clothes suitable for the occasion.

    Rating: 0 = no problems in any area; 1 = problems in one area; 2 = problems in two areas; 3 = problems in three or four areas; 4 = problems in five or six areas.

Name ....
Date   ....

0 1 2 3 4

1. General behaviour
    A. Appearance
    B. Non-productive behaviour
    C. Activity level (hypoactive or hyperactive)
    D. Expression
    E. Responsibility
    F. Punctuality
    G. Reality orientation

    Subtotal

2. *Interpersonal behaviour*
    A. Independence
    B. Co-operation
    C. Self-assertion (compliant or dominant)
    D. Sociability
    E. Attention-getting behaviour
    F. Negative response from others

    Subtotal

3. *Task behaviour*
    A. Engagement
    B. Concentration
    C. Co-ordination
    D. Follow directions
    E. Activity neatness or attention to detail
    F. Problem-solving
    G. Complexity and organisation of task
    H. Initial learning
    I. Interest in activity
    J. Interest in accomplishment
    K. Decision making
    L. Frustration tolerance

    Subtotal

Scale: 0 = normal, 1 = minimal, 2 = mild, 3 = moderate, 4 = severe.

Comments

Therapist's signature ....

Figure 4.3 COTE scale.

The form has been designed for flexible usage being an observation checklist a record of performance over time and an actual report which goes into the medical notes (providing other team members understand the references).

The Volitional Questionnaire (de las Heras, 1995)
This questionnaire arises from the model of human occupation and was developed to assess volition in people with chronic mental health problems or with learning disabilities (i.e. people who have limitations in cognitive or verbal abilities). The assessment involves observing the person in different activity sessions in terms of fourteen volitional indicators related to: (a) intrinsic motivation, (b) personal causation and (c) values/interests. The patient/client is rated along a four-point scale (passive, hesitant, involved or spontaneous) for each indicator. Examples of rated item are: 'Spontaneously demonstrates interest/curiosity in the environment' and 'Is hesitant about trying new things'.

The strength of this assessment is that it offers a reasonably simple, systematic way of observing aspects of volition and motivation – a significant problem for this patient/client group. As with all observational tools therapists have to make inferences which could reduce its reliability. Given some therapists' idiosyncratic scoring patterns, it is not yet known whether reliability can be achieved without special training. A further limitation is that there is a ceiling effect for clients with higher volition (Chern *et al.*, 1996). Its research base is still developing and further revisions may take place, though early indications are that it has been positively received.

The Volitional Questionnaire and User's manual (which includes two useful case simulations) can be obtained from: Model of Human Occupation Clearinghouse, Department of Occupational Therapy, University of Illinois at Chicago, 1919 West Taylor Street, Chicago, IL 60657, USA.

ACIS – The Assessment of Communication and Interaction Skills (Forsyth, 1995)
The ACIS is an observational assessment which aims to gather data on the communication and interaction skills displayed during occupational/social situations (e.g. a cooking group). Three domains are assessed consisting of 20 action verbs/skills to observe, i.e.

- Physicality (e.g. contacts – makes physical contact with others; gazes – uses eyes to communicate and interact with others).
- Information exchange (e.g. articulates – produces clear, understandable speech).
- Relations (e.g. collaborates – co-ordinates one's own action with others toward a common end goal).

The manual offers full details about the standard scoring system used for each action verb. For example, a score of 2 for information exchange implies: 'ineffective ability asserting which impacts on social action; seems to procrastinate, be stubborn, get in others' way; has difficulty making effort for self; speaks with some confidence but also with some doubt; uses indirect approach with others which causes delay in social action; and makes requests without being specific which causes delay in social situation'.

This assessment was initially developed by Simon (1989), further developed/validated by Salamy (1993) and extensively revised by Forsyth (1995) who was helped by 52 Scottish occupational therapists!

Preliminary research on this newly developed assessment suggest a good level of validity and reliability aided by the detailed action verb measures. Appropriately, the assessment manual emphasises the need to observe patients/clients in meaningful situations and how therapists should assess the behaviour in terms of the social and cultural context. Whilst it takes time to get used to the jargon and use of terms, the meanings are spelt out well and familiarity brings ease.

The manual containing research to date, rating guidelines and score sheet, can be purchased from: Model of Human Occupation Clearinghouse, University of Illinois at Chicago, 1919 West Taylor Street, Chicago, IL 60657, USA.

Self-rating methods

These assessments involve the patient/client in formally completing a rating scale or questionnaire (or similar). The self-rating method is used in a variety of ways and can measure patients'/clients' own perceptions of themselves, their attitudes, feelings or their interests.

Aims

Self-rating assessments aim to explore the person's own view of their world. Often used in conjunction with counselling interviews, they can act as a tool to promote insight and self-awareness.

Recording something in black and white can be more powerful than simply saying it. To illustrate this consider the person who ticks a box saying she would like to have a work role in the future. She is admitting it is a possibility and as it is recorded, she cannot deny having said it. Simply saying 'I might like to have a job in the future' can be taken as a throw away line and forgotten.

Self-rating assessments can help with patients'/clients' motivation for treatment. For one thing, they are actively involved in identifying their needs/problem areas. However, more than that, some people enjoy filling out questionnaires (perhaps they remind us of the fun self-scoring quizzes which regularly crop up in popular magazines!).

Application

Self rating methods can be used on their own or (more commonly) used as a tool as part of a wider interview/discussion process. Some forms cover more factual material and can be easily/quickly filled out by patients/clients (e.g. forms which relate to address; type of dwelling; home circumstances or simply interest checklists). Other forms are more complex and may be best discussed with the patient/client. For instance, with a Role Checklist, some people may be unclear about the term 'role' or feel unable to determine what category their roles come under. They may want to explore their feelings/attitudes before committing themselves to putting something down in writing.

The following excerpts from four different assessments (which focus respectively on hobbies, work, social anxiety and self-concept) nicely illustrate the range of self-rating assessments available.

Hobby interest checklist
Please tick the activities which interest you most:

☐ pottery
☐ dressmaking
☐ woodwork
☐ watching television
☐ play
☐ reading
☐ gardening
☐ sport
☐ cooking
☐ typing
☐ ...

Note that this type of form is often best used in the early stages of treatment, where a lot of information can be recorded, stored and possibly used towards planning treatment. They are forms which can easily be filled out by the patient/client to cover 'factual' information quickly. Care must be taken not to dehumanise the process by reducing the person's view of themselves to a few ticks. Thus some discussion after the person has completed the form will increase its value.

Work assessment form (weekly record)
Apply rating criteria of 0 = no serious problems, 1 = some problems, 2 = definite problems needing further help.

Skill area	Patient rating	Staff rating	Comments
accuracy			
speed			
neatness			
organisation			
coping with pressure			
...			

Note that this is an example of an ongoing evaluation form where the patient is actively monitoring his or her own performance in co-operation with the therapist. The aim of this method is to increase the individual's awareness and involvement, therefore improving motivation. If a large discrepancy between the patient's and therapist's score arises, that can be interesting in itself or it may highlight the need for further observations. This type of form is perhaps best used on a regular basis (e.g. during weekly interviews) with the same therapist providing a consistent standard to measure any improvements.

Social anxiety rating scale
Select the choice of difficulty which most closely fits how you feel about the following social situations: 0 = no difficulty, 1 = slight difficulty, 2 = moderate difficulty, 3 = great difficulty, 4 = avoid area.

Situation	*Rating/date*	*Rating/date*
going to parties		
going into restaurants		
meeting strangers		
initiating a conversation		
maintaining a conversation		
…		

Note that this is an example of a behavioural rating scale which could be used prior to social skills training. Its value lies in how it specifically pinpoints the person's problem areas. As the material is potentially emotive, care needs to be taken on presenting this to a patient/client. It is perhaps best used within a counselling-type interview, where answers can be expanded on and discussed. If the questionnaire can be filled out honestly (given a safe therapeutic relationship), then it can act as a valuable baseline to which the individual concerned can subsequently refer (hopefully confirming progress!).

Self-concept questionnaire
Please circle the appropriate answer. I would like to learn …

that I am a person of worth and value	yes	no
to be less self-destructive	yes	no
to feel better about my appearance	yes	no
to feel I am competent	yes	no
to be more assertive …	yes	no

Note that a range of self-rating tools like the one above have been designed in an attempt to grapple with patients'/clients' views of themselves and their emotional responses. They are particularly valuable for promoting insight, and can be useful when comparing the person's own view with that of others. Given their nature they are potentially threatening, and are certainly not easy to complete. At the very least people may have difficulty with the jargon, or in confining abstract concepts to yes/no responses. Moreover, patients/clients may not be ready to apply such concepts to themselves (e.g. may lack the insight). Given these potential pitfalls, much care must be taken both in choosing patients who would find this technique useful, and in presenting it to them in a caring, sensitive way. Often the tests are best used within ongoing counselling sessions or as part of a personal 'diary' in which an individual monitors his or her own feelings more privately.

Summary

To summarise, a range of self-rating questionnaires/forms exist which are adaptable in how they can be used by both therapist and patient. They can act as: (a) a motivator, where the person can be active in his or her own treatment, (b) a casual checklist to touch on verbally or in writing, (c) a vehicle for further discussion/counselling, (d) written evidence to refer back on as treatment progresses, (e) a tool to promote insight and awareness and (f) an opportunity to explore the individual's own view of the world compared to that of others. Whatever type of self-rating method is used, care must be taken not to dehumanise the process and reduce our patient's/client's view of their world to a few ticks. Further, as with any method involving personal reflection, some people may feel threatened or become distressed in the process. A self-rating assessment can be a powerful tool and needs to be presented in a caring, sensitive way.

Published tools

Interest Checklist (Kielhofner and Neville, 1983)

This checklist was originally devised by Matsutsuyu (1969) and then revised by others including Kielhofner and Neville. This is a self-rating tool which requires the person to rate 68 different activities or areas of interest (e.g. gardening, sewing/needlework, playing cards, foreign languages and church activities) according to: (a) level of interest in the past 10 years/past year, (b) whether or not he/she currently participates and (c) if he/she wishes to pursue it in the future.

This assessment is a valuable tool (particularly when combined with discussion) for identifying patterns of interest, as it offers such a comprehensive checklist. It has also been extensively used in clinical research studies (see Kielhofner, 1995). Therapists practicing in the UK may wish to modify the tool by translating some of the American words (such as 'visiting' and 'yardwork') and adding some others (like DIY, horse racing and cricket!).

The (modified) Interest Checklist is available from: The National Institute of Health, Occupational Therapy Department, Building 10, Room 65235, Bethesda, MD 20892, USA.

Role Checklist (Oakley, 1981)

This checklist is a self-rating form designed to obtain information about the types of roles a person engages in (comparing past, present and future roles). The checklist describes 10 roles (student, worker, volunteer, caregiver, home maintainer, friend, family member, religious participant, hobbyist/amateur and participant in organisations).The significance of these roles for the person are then rated (e.g. not at all valuable, somewhat valuable and very valuable).

The checklist is a valuable simple tool (particularly when used in conjunction with discussion – at least to explain what 'role' is!) for understanding the person's own perceptions of their life roles and can be applied in many situations. Information about congruence or mismatch of roles regarding frequency of performance versus their value can be highly significant (for instance if a person does not value the carer role yet performs it frequently or vice versa). With its concentrated focus on occupational roles, it has become a popular tool for occupational therapists around the world. Research carried out when it was first developed suggests reasonable validity and reliability (Oakley *et al.*, 1986).

Occupational Questionnaire (Smith, Kielhofner and Watts, 1986)

This questionnaire is a self-rating tool where patients/clients describe their typical use of time (activities carried out are listed for every half an hour). The person then rates each activity on a Likert-type scale according to: (a) whether it is work, daily living, recreation or rest, (b) how competently he/she does it, (c) how important it is and (d) how much it is enjoyed. A variety of scores can be calculated to give an insight into the person's pattern of occupational activity.

The strength of this tool is its focus on occupational activities and the insights it yields about the person's own view of how he/she copes. This questionnaire can be applied in a variety of treatment settings and it can be useful for understanding the needs of different types of patients/clients (including individuals with physical problems). The process of filling it out can feel laborious for patients/clients, but it offers a clear cut account of the person's daily life activities and any changes can be simply measured. This assessment has been used extensively in clinical research studies in the US.

The guide is available from: Model of Human Occupation Clearinghouse, University of Illinois at Chicago, 1919 West Taylor Street, Chicago, IL 60657, USA.

COPM – Canadian Occupational Performance Measure (Law et al., 1994)

The COPM combines interview and self-rating measures whilst maintaining a client-centred focus. Questions are asked about: (a) self-care (personal care, functional mobility, community management), (b) productivity (paid/unpaid work, household management, play/school) and (c) leisure (quiet recreation, active research, socialisation). When the patient/client identifies a problem area, he or she is asked to rate/weight its importance (scale of 1–10). Then the person is asked to choose the five most important problems and rate them in terms of performance and satisfaction. A numerical score is then calculated.

The strength of this assessment is its focus on the patient's/client's own values and view of their occupational performance. Its concentrated focus on occupational performance has made it a popular new tool for occupational therapists, particularly those concerned with physical and practical problems. Whilst the validity of the subjective response scores can be questioned, they are meaningful for comparison on reassessment. Research evaluating its clinical utility (Toomey, Nicholson and Carswell, 1995) highlights some other limitations. For instance, clients need to have a reasonable level of insight/cognitive skills and some therapists find the assessment uncomfortable and time consuming to use. The number of clinical research studies (e.g. Waters, 1995) using this measure is growing.

The assessment can be obtained from: The Canadian Association of Occupational Therapists, 110 Eglinton Avenue West, 3rd floor, Toronto, Ontario, Canada, M4R 1A3. A number of training videos about this assessment and the Canadian client-centred model of occupational performance have been produced. They are available from: Canadian Association of Occupational Therapists, Carleton Training and Technology Centre, Suite 3400, 1125 Colonel by Drive, Ottawa, Ontario, Canada, K1S 5R1.

Psychodynamic activities

Activities employed within the psychodynamic framework are designed to tap deeper feelings and unconscious material. Any creative activity could be employed – the key point being how well the activity facilitates self-expression and allows an exploration of feelings/unconscious motivations.

Application

Psychodynamic activities rely heavily on the interpretive and analytical skills of the therapist. Since their conception they have been adapted and remoulded to suit the needs of various therapies. In the United States some projective tests have been published and semi-standardised, such as the Azima Battery and the Shoemeyen Battery (Hemphill, 1982, pp. 57–86). Whilst occupational therapists in the UK do not generally use formal projective tests, we have taken some of their principles and devised a range of psychodynamic activities that can be used for assessment purposes. These activities provide us with a wealth of information about the feelings, needs and hopes of an individual. The following activities are ones most commonly employed in the UK.

Projective art

Any activity can be used projectively. One example is painting on two halves of a paper: 'an aspect of myself I dislike' and 'an aspect of myself I like'. Not surprisingly, people with a low self-esteem find the latter task, of acknowledging something they like about themselves, difficult. As such, this is also a useful exercise in therapy, and occasionally the therapist may have to insist that both sides of the paper are completed. If done in a group, this kind of exercise can also greatly aid self-exploration, particularly when parallels are drawn between the group members.

Creative writing

Any creative writing activity can be used. As one example, imagine the wealth of personal information which could be revealed by writing 'A friend's description of me' or 'A conversation with my pet if he could talk'. Such activities attempt to elicit a self-view which is more difficult to write in the first person. It can also be valuable to reflect on others' view of oneself.

Playtherapy

Observing a child playing freely can reveal much about his or her inner world. Commonly, a doll's house can be used to explore family dynamics. A point of interesting debate that arises in this method is whether or not everything the child plays out has a meaning. Whilst psychodynamic theory would say 'yes', pointing to symbolic meanings, I feel we should not be so dogmatic. Instead, we can say that sometimes a child's play can be extremely revealing, with the play being either a reflection of family life or a form of wish-fulfilment.

Diary

Patients/clients might be asked to keep a diary of their feelings, reactions and behaviours in the context of general life happenings. The process of writing a diary can offer insights to both the patient/client and therapist. It can be particularly useful for people on controlled drinking or eating programmes where they use the diary to record their consumption and make links between their behaviour and feelings. Lacey (1984), for example, recommends such an approach when treating women suffering bulimia nervosa.

THEORY INTO PRACTICE

Case example: **Selecting and combining assessments**

The following case examples detail one therapist's choice of assessments for different individuals. Do you agree with the selections?

1. Ann, a housewife, aged 56, is depressed, labile and says she is a failure. Assessment methods selected: (a) counselling interview using Role Checklist, (b) Occupational Questionnaire and (c) a self-concept self-rating questionnaire.
2. Thomas, aged 76, has a possible diagnosis of dementia and some mobility problems. Assessment methods selected: (a) AMPS, (b) CAPE, and (c) home visit observing mobility and the environment.
3. Leroy, aged 45, suffers from chronic schizophrenia. He lacks drive/motivation and has poor functional skills. Assessment methods selected: (a) Volitional Questionnaire (using cooking, painting and printing activities), (b) Interest Checklist and (c) FPR.
4. Jamie, a boy of 8, with an apparently deprived childhood, has been referred because of destructive behaviour. Assessment methods selected: (a) observation of free play in a one-to-one session, (b) projective art, 'draw your family', and (c) observation in structured small group activity (e.g. cookery).
5. Susan, aged 30, is recovering from a manic depressive episode and has been referred to occupational therapy to prepare for discharge. Assessment methods selected: (a) OCAIRS, (b) observation using COTE scale and (c) ACIS.
6. Pat, aged 45, has multiple functional problems resulting from the neurological

damage sustained in a head injury. Assessment methods selected: (a) COPM, (b) OPHI and (c) COTNAB.
7. John, a 30-year-old man with a learning disability is being resettled in a new community house from his parents' home. Assessment methods selected: (a) ABS, (b) Life Experience checklist and (c) domestic assessment.

4.3 DEBATES ABOUT ASSESSMENT – SOME PERSONAL REFLECTIONS

In this chapter I have implicitly advocated the use of fairly *formal* and specifically focused assessments, over *informal* and unstructured methods. The therapists who primarily support more formalised methods argue: (a) specifically focused assessments promote a clearer understanding of particular issues/needs, (b) the effect of our own biases, values, idiosyncrasies can be reduced by adopting standard routines, (c) focused assessments facilitate more focused treatment, (d) patients/clients (to say nothing about other team members) often trust and respond better to procedures which are perceived as 'professional', and (e) the stronger the research base backing the assessment, the more credibility it has as a tool – arguably essential in these days of performance indicators and outcome measures.

On the other hand, the therapists who support the more intuitive, unstructured ways of assessing patients would argue: (a) 'Standardised assessments are too artificial, cold, mechanical and patients get overly stressed when they know they are being tested', (b) 'The important thing is to get on and treat patients. We don't have the time to do all these assessments' and (c) 'Some of these assessments are very judgemental. Do we have the right to make such judgements when we hardly know the person?'

In this section some of these debates will be aired, acknowledging their wisdoms, whilst challenging their assumptions.

Science obscuring art?

Picture the following situation. An occupational therapist is observing how a patient manages a task without prompting/assistance. The patient makes a mistake, feels confused and inadequate, and becomes stressed, then fails in the task. The occupational therapist does not intervene and simply records the result. Can this be right? Is occupational therapy in danger of losing its essentially humanistic values in bowing towards the pressure of science? What justification is there to put a patient under stress in the name of objective data?

I would certainly agree that we need to remember 'the person' behind the 'subject to be assessed'. It seems to me that this therapist could well have forgotten that assessment is part of treatment. We must not destroy the 'art' of maintaining a therapeutic relationship in the name of 'science'.

However, perhaps we are being grossly unfair to the scientists, who also support the need to maintain a rapport with their subjects. In the situation of a task assessment where it would be important not to intervene (and therefore skew the findings), the good, scientific therapist would take care to be supportive – both before and after, if not during the test. The patient/client needs to understand the assessment situation (where possible) and should know what he or she and the therapist are doing, and why. The therapist should be flexible enough to jettison the task if it is creating undue problems – another form of assessment may be more appropriate at that time.

In debate I would also raise another point which is that the prime purpose of assessment is to gather information which will ultimately help the patient/client by enabling more effective treatment to be planned. In this case, the more secure we are about the accuracy of that information, the better. However, each clinical situation is different – in each situation we may need to find a different balance between 'science' (where we aim to be systematic and ensure accuracy) or 'art' (where we lean towards more creative, intuitive approaches).

Published tools or home-grown?

Are published assessments better? In this age of quality assurance and measurable outcomes should we stop using homegrown methods? My own view is that any assessment is only a 'tool'. It should be used selectively and judiciously in whatever way is most beneficial. Ideally therapists should become familiar with, and experiment with, different assessments and thus make an informed choice.

Published assessments have the value that they have been tried, tested and researched. This strong research base carries with it a number of benefits. First, these are often professionally packaged, containing special equipment and detailed instructions for carrying out the assessment. Secondly, it can be useful to compare one's own use of the assessment with findings from other clinical studies. Thirdly, it can be important to know levels of validity and inter-rater reliability. Finally, published assessments often carry more weight and are respected by other team members. I know some doctors who will not look at results if they are measured by unpublished and non-standardised assessments(!).

Of course (in common with all types of assessments) they have their limitations. For one thing, the published tool may only be relevant for a particular patient/client group. At a broader level, any assessment will have its own cultural bias (a criticism often levelled by UK practioners at the terminology and ideas contained within some US publications). No assessment should be blindly adhered to or its value assumed simply because it has been published or standardised.

Homegrown tools have the value that they are locally developed so may be more appropriate for specific local needs. We need to use our own professional judgement to decide which assessment to use and in what context.

Best use of scarce resources?

A common complaint given against assessment is 'we do not have the time or staffing available to do extensive one-to-one assessments'. This reality is a large stumbling block. At the risk of answering glibly, however, it would seem to be about choice of priorities. Do we prefer to treat more patients, do less assessment and run the risk of supplying vague treatment? Or do we prefer to assess each patient in order to ensure some degree of individual treatment planning? At all points of treatment we have to make choices about priorities. It may well be impractical to consider lengthy in-depth assessments for every patient. Therefore, it makes sense to:

1. Select only the patients/clients who seem to be at an appropriate stage for the kind of occupational therapy available. Reports from other team members are useful here.
2. Select the most useful assessment method to use, given the patient's/client's skills, problem areas, and the therapist's abilities.
3. Select the area on which occupational therapy should focus specifically. This is where the team needs to work together (e.g. the nurse focusing on personal care skills while the occupational therapist considers the home environment and the social worker considers family support).

Another question I have heard posed in this context concerns the possible dangers of spending too many resources on assessment whilst never getting down to treatment. I would agree that there is a danger of occupational therapists 'over-assessing' – spotting the problems without considering problem solving. This may be a result of therapists feeling assessment is a clear, valuable role; therefore, they develop their skills in this area and so treatment time is diminished. It is worth considering this further, however. Isn't assessment part of treatment? A key part of interviewing, for example, can be the use of counselling techniques. Also the deeper one-to-one contact of intensive assessment may have more remedial benefit than longer 'treatment' consisting of being in a large, more casual group. In the end, the only justification for assessment is when specific recommendations for treatment or follow-up elsewhere are made.

Making judgements

Therapists commonly experience some tensions when making evaluations of their patient's/client's performance. Often the evaluations are crucial – involving major quality of life decisions. For instance, a person's discharge may be dependent on the therapist's decision concerning a safety/risk assessment.

Such 'power' can sit uncomfortably on our shoulders. Do we have the right to make judgements about patients – particularly on the basis of one or two formal assessments? My view is that we have to make judgements – they cannot be avoided. However, the judgements we make should be contained within the limits of 'professional requirements' and not jaundiced by our personal moral standards, religious beliefs or political views. Whilst we are entitled to have and advocate these, we should not subject others to them.

How we make professional judgements is an issue of immediate practical importance. The following are some pointers towards making judgements more effective and constructive.

1. Be as *objective* as possible so as to limit the possibility of being blinded by stereotyped perceptions. Here we especially need to guard against being swayed by any labels, diagnosis, etc., which could act as self-fulfilling prophesies (e.g. when working with institutionalised patients, reducing aims to the lowest common denominator). The debate of whether or not we read patients'/clients' case notes prior to the initial meeting is particularly pertinent here. It is probably an individual choice according to how swayed we might be. I personally prefer to form my own initial impression of the person prior to reading the notes. A brief report from the other team members first (e.g. asking if there are any precautions I need to be aware of) is a possible compromise.

2. Acknowledge any gaps or *limitations in your judgements* to avoid possible misinterpretation. An example here is: 'Mary is safe using our department cooker. Further assessment is required to confirm her safety at home'.

3. Devote more energy to *collecting data rather than making inferences*. For example, consider the situation of seeing a person cry. We could fall into making all sorts of interpretations, for instance that he or she is inadequate or being manipulative (see Figure 4.4). Therapists need to take care to avoid over-inferring or interpreting without adequate evidence.

4. Constantly *monitor judgements/assessments* to confirm, deny or adjust to changing circumstances. Here the team can well use each other by sharing impressions on the basis of a person's 24-hour day. Certainly we need to be wary of making firm judgements on the basis of limited evidence. Using only one or two tests is potentially problematic unless we limit the scope of the information we are trying to gain.

5. Acknowledge any *assumptions* about what is 'normal' or 'desired behaviour', which may underlie our judgements. This is particularly important over time as views and fashions change. If a patient is behaving promiscuously, do we assess this as his/her habitual pattern or a sign of a hyperactive mental state? Also we each have our own cultural standards which may be highly relevant. A good illustration of this is a person who eats with their fingers who is assessed as being disinhibited and confused, when this is in fact his or her normal practice.

The experience of being assessed

Sometimes as therapists we can become blasé about the assessment process. It is such a routine part of our work we can forget how difficult – even traumatic – it is

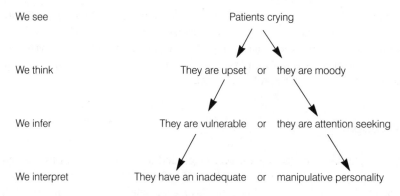

Figure 4.4 Different interpretations of data.

for some patients/clients. Understandably, people can feel nervous about their performance and test results – all the more so if they recognise possible implications, for instance that discharge will be postponed. Other people may find the assessment process itself threatening. We are so accustomed to receiving personal details from others that we may forget how difficult and painful self-disclosure can be. As therapists we need to be sensitive to these different reactions and try to offer both empathy and explanations. We should feel honoured and humble when someone shares something of themselves and not simply resent it when he or she is defensive. Also results may need to be fed back to the person carefully.

This then raises other questions about how to present the assessment process to our patients/clients. If the assessment is going to generate undue tensions, could we not observe unobtrusively? Clearly there is no definitive answer here as it depends on the individual concerned and the team approach. In general, we can fall back on our professional-legal responsibility where we are under continuing pressure to allow 'consumers' access to reports and to be informed about treatment. The professional-moral argument would emphasise the need to collaborate with our patients/clients in treatment planning. Maintaining a 'professional silence' or finding devious ways to uncover problems works against encouraging mutual trust.

If a patient/client is overly threatened or anxious on being observed or assessed, we need to consider the situation further. A number of factors may be involved. First, the patient/client may feel that he or she is being judged negatively. Here the problem would seem to lie more with how the therapist is presenting assessment in the first place. Alternatively, the person may feel a certain amount of natural performance tension on being given set tasks. We must take this into account, of course, and consider his or her performance in several contexts, over time. Lastly, we may be inadvertently appearing too distant or threatening, e.g. by our non-verbal behaviour. The writing of notes during assessments is an example of this, and whilst it may be perfectly acceptable, or even desirable, it has a negative side if human contact is broken.

I believe that wherever possible our patients/clients should have some control over what information is gleaned from assessment, and how. They need to be encouraged to alert us to what is important to them, and what they wish us to know. As always, a good place to start in our thinking is to consider how we would like to be treated given a similar situation.

CONCLUSION

This chapter has covered a great deal of ground about the range of assessments available and the implications of applying them in practice. Five different assessment methods and their applications have been analysed. Each one has been shown to have both strengths and limitations (see Table 4.1 for a summary evaluation), and, as such, often we will use several methods in combination.

In the last analysis any assessment remains a 'tool' for an occupational therapist to use – a tool which should be applied selectively, judiciously and sensitively. The best assessors are the ones who remember they are also therapists. The best assessments are the ones which occur as part of a wider therapeutic process.

Once the therapist has begun to build a relationship with the patient/client and preliminary assessment findings are established, the therapist is ready to start planning treatment – the subject we turn to in the next chapter.

Discussion questions

1. To what extent is assessment a part of treatment?
2. What is the value of using a standardised or published assessment over a home-grown tool?
3. What are the strengths and limitations of each method of assessment?
4. Should patients/clients know when they are being assessed and why?
5. What is meant by reliability and validity, and why are these important?
6. Explain how various psychological theories are implicit within each assessment method.

Table 4.1 Summary evaluation of types of assessments and their application

Type	Main focus of assessment	Value/strengths	Limitations/weaknesses	Implications for use
Standardised tests	Occupational performance and behaviour; cognitive/perceptual/social/motor skills.	Scientific rigour; validity/reliability increased. More 'official' so often respected by colleagues and patients/clients. Baseline for research.	Can be impersonal and anxiety provoking. Value lost if incorrectly applied. May not have local relevance. Assessor may need special training.	Strict adherence to standard practice important. Times before and after testing important for explanations, relationship building, and feedback. Use norms relevant for that patient/client group
Interview	Life situation, self-perception, attitudes, interests, behaviour, mood.	Individuals can communicate what they feel is important. Relationship building eased. Factual and subjective aspects can be covered.	Responses often depend on skill of therapist regarding: being sensitive/listening and asking the right questions. People can lie. People may not be skilled verbally or too withdrawn to talk.	Be clear about the aims of the interview – particularly as the patient/client may well go through several interviews. Develop skills of active listening.
Structured observation	Skills, behaviour, task performance, group interaction.	Judgements made on the basis of what is seen, not on inferences or assurances from patient/client – therefore fairly objective. More practical/activity based so fits our role.	Validity/reliability not assured as it relies on therapist observation skills and accurate interpretation. Limited contexts for observation. Subjective experience is not so easily identified.	Consider using structured forms and tasks in preference to general observation. Recognise limitations and continue to develop skills. Draw on observations at different times and situations.

Self-rating methods	Feelings, attitudes, interests, self concept and factual information.	Taps more abstract material and subjective experience. Person can communicate what he or she feels is important. Respects person's capacity and responsibility for treatment.	People can lie. Process can be impersonal. Certain forms may threaten, irritate or be too abstract.	Use the forms as a vehicle for patient's/client's growth and development. Be flexible with how they are applied, e.g. some people may wish to fill it out privately and then discuss it.
	Feelings, attitudes, self concept, relationships, unconscious material.	Taps more abstract and unconscious material.	Therapist's level of skill with the medium and interpretations crucial.	Feelings expressed must be dealt with, not just assessed – so the process may take time.
Psychodynamic activities		Can assist with relationship building. Can be therapeutic in itself (e.g. increasing insight).	Can be emotionally threatening, painful or contradindi-cated.	Avoid interpretations – or at least seek confirmation from the patient/client. Patients/clients and activities need to be selected carefully.

Planning treatment 5

Planning treatment is a process involving the organisation of information in such a way that the patient's/client's problems are identified, treatment principles are specified and treatment goals/activities negotiated. It is a *logical* procedure where aims of treatment follow from problems identified. It can also be an exercise in *creativity* where, in the design of treatment, we consider a wide range of possible ways of enhancing a patient's/client's functioning, before agreeing a treatment plan. In essence this involves three stages:

- *Organising the information* – information obtained from assessments is organised to highlight problems and priority areas.
- *Establishing aims, goals and objectives* – considering both short- and long-term aspects.
- *Designing the programme* – grading the activity, therapist role and environment to meet aims.

Whilst these stages look straightforward, they are not. A multiplicity of interacting factors need to be taken into account at each point. Further, each stage often requires a complex negotiation between the therapist, treatment team and patient/client. This chapter will begin to explore some of these complexities, discussing each stage of treatment planning in turn. A final section will offer some case illustrations of different levels of treatment planning.

5.1 ORGANISING THE INFORMATION

There are four tasks involved in organising our assessment information: (a) processing the information, (b) identifying the problem, (c) identifying positive aspects and (d) selecting the priority problem.

Processing the information

Planning within a team context

In the initial stages of planning treatment we need to process a considerable volume of information arising from the occupational therapy assessment findings and the other team members' reports. In addition factors regarding the practicalities of treatment need to be considered. Table 5.1 summarises the range of information which needs to be taken into account.

Table 5.1 Range of information

Occupational therapy findings	*Team members' reports*	*Practical aspects*
• General functioning of person	• Clinical condition and prognosis	• Limits on treatment
• Expected environment	• Past and present treatment	such as time and
• Social, domestic, work circumstances and lifestyle	• Social history	resources available
• Skills and interests		

In terms of the *occupational therapy findings*, we are concerned to analyse the person's: (a) general functioning, (b) social, domestic and work roles, circumstances and general lifestyle, (c) expected environment (e.g. how much support is available), and (d) skills, interests and positive aspects which can be used in the treatment (see Figure 4.1).

In terms of *team member reports*, we would take note of the patient's/client's clinical condition and prognosis; past and present treatment; and social history. Ideally the team would discuss a division of labour whereby different team members would focus on different issues (for instance the nurses might work on self-care, the doctor communicates with the family whilst the occupational therapist explores work options).

Alongside processing clinical priorities, we take into account *practical aspects* such as resources, time and treatment opportunities available. It may well be necessary to compromise. For instance, if a patient is likely to be discharged quickly, it may be more relevant to activate community support systems rather than become involved in treatment which would have to be curtailed.

Focusing on priorities

For the occupational therapist, some parts of this information is more relevant than other parts of it. In-depth knowledge about the diagnosis, for example, is interesting but less important than a recognition of how the disorder is affecting the patient's/client's functioning. Again, past medical and psychiatric history is of less concern to occupational therapists, than is recognising their 'expected environment', which will influence future roles and needs.

THEORY INTO PRACTICE

Use and limits of diagnosis

Occupational therapists try to avoid depersonalising labels and blanket diagnoses, recognising that illness is only one aspect of the whole person. Two main dangers of employing diagnosis are: (a) it takes us down a medical model route, which focuses us unduly on the course of illness rather than on coping/health which is more in tune with occupational therapy philosophy, and (b) stereotyping people can result in stereotyped treatment where an individual's needs are disregarded.

However, diagnosis does have a role to play in our work. First, knowing a person's diagnosis gives us clues about the likely *course*, *prognosis* and *contraindications* of that particular condition. Armed with this information, our clinical judgement and long-term aims will be more realistic. Secondly, we need to know about diagnoses in order to *work with others* in the treatment team who do use diagnosis as a starting point. This is particularly true in acute in-patient settings where much discussion will take place along medical model lines. Thirdly, some therapists may play a role in the team determining *differential diagnoses*. In principle, however, our focus is on functioning and occupational performance, not the person's illness.

The process of clinical reasoning

The process of organising the information is a complex one and involves more than simply rational problem analysis. The therapist employs a range of mental strategies and cognitive processes (that are simultaneously creative, intuitive and logical) to build an understanding of the individual concerned. An interpersonal dimension is also present where the therapist engages with the patient/client to decide upon and implement treatment. This whole process is often referred to in the literature as **clinical reasoning**.

Exactly how clinical reasoning occurs is the subject of much debate. A growing pool of literature reflects diverse, often conflicting, accounts on how professionals think.* The point on which everyone seems agreed is recognising that our thinking is complex and multi-dimensional. The Theory into Practice box below selectively outlines four of the more widely discussed types of clinical reasoning.

---

*For those readers who wish to grapple with the richness of debates I recommend the following sources: Mattingly (1991), Fleming (1991), Mattingly and Fleming (1994) and Shell and Cervero (1993) in the US; and Ryan (1995) and Munroe (1995) in the UK. See also the special Clinical Reasoning Issue in the *British Journal of Occupational Therapy* (May, 1996).

THEORY INTO PRACTICE

Four types of clinical reasoning

Type	Description	Example
Scientific reasoning (e.g. Rogers, 1983)	Systematic, logical thinking process based on hypothesis testing, scientific model making, plus use of research-based theory and techniques.	Therapist formulates problems based on knowledge of patient's condition and the results of a standardised assessment.
Narrative reasoning (e.g. Mattingly, 1991)	Phenomenological process where stories are used to understand an individual's meanings – thinking involves empathy, improvisation and attention to values/beliefs.	Therapist and patient share their pictures of how the individual experiences his or her disability – they look at past, present and future scenarios.
Interactive reasoning (e.g. Fleming, 1991)	Reasoning arises out of the interaction between therapist and patient/client – the therapist acts on subtle cues in order to motivate and engage the individual in treatment.	Therapist modifies approach during treatment session to relieve some of the patient's tension, e.g. by lightening the interaction with some humour and small talk.
Pragmatic reasoning (e.g. Schell and Cervero, 1993)	The socio-cultural context, setting and practical/environmental constraints, plus therapist's own life experiences, all influence clinical decision making.	Therapist plans a patient's discharge programme which takes into account limited home support and day care provision.

Identifying the problems

Occupational therapists treat people who have a multiplicity of problems. Emotional, cognitive, physical, social and functional problems are usually intertwined in complex ways. The process of understanding these problems is made more difficult because of the subjective way individuals experience them. A large problem to one person, may be irrelevant to others. For example, one person may be devastated by losing their job, whereas another person might accept this phlegmatically. It is vital that therapists understand the underlying and dynamic nature of our patients'/clients' problems if we are to treat them effectively. To begin to explore some of these complexities, three different ways occupational therapists approach problems are discussed below.

Function not illness

When a person becomes ill or stressed, their ability to function in daily life is impaired. Occupational therapists focus on these functional aspects as opposed to the illness itself. For example, take two people with different diagnoses, one of schizophrenia and the other of depression. From our point of view they may well display similar functional problems where their daily occupational performance is affected by being withdrawn, apathetic and passive. They may both have stopped looking after themselves so their self-care is poor. They may both tend to sit around all day doing nothing – having few interests and difficulties in relating to others. They are both likely to have reduced task performance skills which impairs their ability to work and a psychiatric history which means future employment is unlikely. They may both require long-term support in the community. These are the functional problems which we would address (see Table 5.2).

Table 5.2 Problems relate to functioning

Problem	Description	Effect on function
Poor task performance	Unable to carry our simple task independently – sequencing a particular problem	Dependent for dressing and self-care routines
Passive, unmotivated behaviour	Does not initiate conversation or activity unless prompted	Socially isolated at home

Focus on the individual in his/her social context

Having recognised that patients/clients may have similar problems, we still try to value the uniqueness of each individual. Each person has his or her own skills, problems, needs and motives. Each person has their own personal history of experiences which are set within a wider social/cultural heritage. Thus each person requires an individualised treatment programme. We might use the same occupational therapy activity with two different people but the treatment process is likely to be very different. Our approach and way of handling each person; the aims of the activity; how it is graded and adapted; and how it fits into the rest of the person's treatment, are all specific to the individual.

Consider the different ways that cooking has been used with the three different people below.

- Annie is a 20-year-old on the point of leaving home. She has been dependent on her family, and lacks both skills and confidence in her ability to cope as an adult. As part of a wider programme of skills training and developing her *sense of personal causation*, Annie learns to cook in occupational therapy.

- Rufus is a 40-year-old man who has been in and out of hospital for years. He is passive and lacks drive to do anything. He enjoys cooking, however, and it provides a useful way to both activate him and *assess his task performance*.
- Meena is 65-year-old socially anxious women. As Meena is a confident cook, the therapist recommends she join a local cookery class with the aim of *encouraging social interaction* in a relatively non-threatening way.

Being realistic

Being realistic means we sometimes have to make difficult choices. We may need to accept that treatment will not result in a 'cure' or full employment, etc. Relapses, deteriorating functioning and the need for life-long medication are real possibilities for many people suffering mental health problems. Therapists need to be realistic (without being unduly pessimistic) as they may be called upon to help a patient/client come to terms with their likely prognosis. Ignoring potential future problems will not help anyone.

It is important to be realistic about what problems we can do something about as opposed to those which are beyond our scope. Consider the case of Winnie.

Winnie is 53 years old and was discharged into a group home from a large mental institution 6 years ago. The group home arrangement broke down within a couple of months. Now Winnie lives on the streets except when it is very cold when she goes into a 'doss house'. She lives by a combination of begging and charity, moving from place to place with her carrier bag of belongings. Her self-care is extremely poor as she has limited opportunities to wash, and she lacks both the awareness and the motivation to be concerned about her appearance and hygiene. Winnie is admitted to hospital several times a year suffering hallucinations/delusions and behaving in a bizarre and aggressive manner. She is usually discharged as soon as possible.

It is hard to admit, but the reality is that we can do little about most of Winnie's problems. For a start, her *social problems* of poverty, homelessness, unemployment and poor health/hygiene are probably intractable. Also, in the current context of 'Community Care' policies there are financial and ideological pressures to discharge people from hospital as soon as possible. Winnie's *self-care problems* are largely a result of her situation. Implementing a self-care programme would be both an imposition of our values and a relatively pointless exercise if she is returning to the streets. Winnie's *psychotic symptoms* are also beyond our scope as only medication can stabilise her mental state. It might be possible for Winnie to be referred to a rehabilitation unit (of which occupational therapy is a part) or a domestic rehabilitation programme could be implemented towards a housing resettlement process. Realistically speaking, this will take many months and Winnie is unlikely to be sufficiently committed to the treatment. In the last analysis, for many reasons, Winnie may not receive or follow through long-term rehabilitation. Arguably our best role is to offer her brief periods of pleasure to enhance her *quality of life* and to act on her behalf as an *advocate*. For instance, we could try to ensure she has some supportive follow-up in the community when she is discharged.

Identify positive aspects

Successful treatment acknowledges the patient's/client's strengths, interests and motivations. Strengths are important as often we use a person's skill in another area to help the problem area (e.g. a creative bent being harnessed to learn a craft in order to improve task skills). At the very least we need to remind the individual (and ourselves) of his or her positive points to help balance our emphasis on problems. Interests should be taken into account as part of appreciating a person's social/cultural background and needs. The process of incorporating strengths and interests usually goes some way to aiding motivation to engage in treatment or activity (a crucial variable if treatment is to be effective). For an illustration of this in action see Case illustration 5.1 on page 124.

THEORY INTO PRACTICE

Finding something positive to work with

Bernie, a patient in a forensic unit, presented some problems for the occupational therapist. He was a large man with a history of extremely violent behaviour (often drug related). On the ward he was aggressive and abusive, particularly when asked to do anything. On first meeting the occupational therapist, Bernie threatened her saying she would regret it if she tried to push him. The therapist replied that he could make his own decisions and offered him (with some trepidation!) an open invitation to come down to the activity room. When he presented himself, she acknowledged him but left him to look around on his own. She noticed he returned several times to look at some model airplanes that had been painted by a patient. Bernie was disparaging and told the therapist they were using the wrong type of paint brush. The next day Bernie brought the therapist a paint brush. She asked him if he could show it to the other patient. Thereafter, Bernie took a positive role of leading the model aeroplane group.

Selecting priority problem(s)

Being realistic and focused

We are rarely able to treat all the problems identified in assessment. First, occupational therapy cannot be a panacea for all ills. Secondly, if we tried for a comprehensive coverage of problems, our treatment would stand in danger of being far too wide ranging. Consider, for example, the chronically institutionalised patient, who has received minimal therapy in recent years. The problem list is likely to be long (possibly encompassing: stooped posture, unkempt appearance, hypoactive and passive behaviour, poor reality orientation, poor social skills, low motivation, poor concentration, difficulties in carrying out tasks, etc.). In the initial stages it would be impossible to work on all of these problems. It is far better to select a particular area for focus. Any success we achieve may then have additional positive benefits, rather like a dominoes effect (e.g. Figure 5.1).

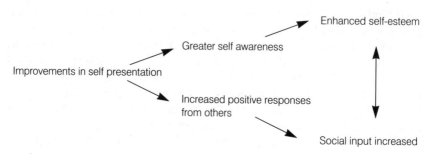

Figure 5.1 Positive benefits of selecting key problems.

Once a person starts to function better in one area, he or she may be able to sort out his or her own situation. We are not responsible for 'fixing' all areas. Take the example of Mick, a 50-year-old ship builder who was made redundant. When he lost his job, he started to drink heavily and suffered marital problems. He spent his time either sitting morosely at home or in the pub. The occupational therapy intervention simply focused on trying to develop some meaningful, productive activities which would positively activate Mick (in his case he enjoyed DIY activities). Treatment was successful. As Mick felt happier, his marital relations improved and he no longer felt the need to abuse alcohol.

Criteria for selecting priorities

The skill of the therapist lies in the selection of a few key problems to work on initially. This can be done on the basis of several criteria:

- Select the most basic or *underlying problem*, e.g. poor social skills may be at the root of the difficulties of a person who is having problems in both relationships and finding/keeping a job.
- The patient/client could be invited to arrange the problem list in a hierarchy. If the patient is working on what he or she *perceives to be important*, then the motivation is likely to be higher.
- The family or staff could select an *initial problem* which they see as over-shadowing all other aspects, e.g. behaviour which is overtly bizarre or out of control often needs to be managed before any fine tuning is attempted.
- The problem which has an *easy solution* could be worked on first, as part of confidence building in the therapist–patient relationship, e.g. teaching relax-

ation techniques for coping with anxiety or supplying a communication aid, immediately.

- Lastly, an important criterion is the influence of whichever *theoretical framework* is being used, e.g. therapists who favour a humanistic approach are more likely to select problems of feelings as being fundamental, whereas behaviourists would direct their attention towards behaviour.

Negotiating the priorities

The therapist's clinical reasoning described above would normally be done in private. At some point, however, the ideas need to be shared and, where possible, explored with the patient/client. Ideally treatment should be negotiated. The patient/client needs to agree the problem or the focus of intervention. For one thing, research (Kleinman *et al.*, 1978 and Cassell *et al.*, 1977, cited in Jenkins *et al.*, 1995) has shown that treatments are more likely to be effective when patients' attitudes and beliefs about disease and treatment are elicited and when the client is enlisted as a therapeutic ally. Jenkins *et al.* describe an interactional approach demonstrating that best practice arises when the therapist invites client participation. If the patient/client is unable to participate, the therapist must be extra concerned to make decisions that are well justified and ethical (Hagedorn, 1995).

THEORY INTO PRACTICE

Example of negotiating the problem

Therapist	During this interview, Jean, you've mentioned a number of problems ranging from what you're feeling inside to the strains of work and home.
Jean	Yes, everywhere I turn there seems to be another problem.
Therapist	(nods, acknowledging Jean's comment) I think we'd find it difficult to work on all those problems at once. Is it possible to narrow them down a bit to see if we can come up with one or two areas to work on first?
Jean	I guess so (unsure).
Therapist	Okay, let's see … which problem causes you the most stress? (The therapist could equally have asked: which problem do you want to get rid of the most? or which problem has the most/least effect on your life?).
Jean	Oh, I don't know …. I can't cope with the children and their screaming …. The biggest problems are at home, I'm so tense …
Therapist	Yes. One of the things we find in therapy is that sometimes, if you get one problem area sorted out, the other problems sort themselves out too. For example, if you were feeling less tense, do you think you might cope with your children's screaming better?

5.2 ESTABLISHING AIMS, GOALS, OBJECTIVES

We now come to the second major stage involved in planning treatment, namely, establishing treatment aims. Once the problem(s) to be worked on have been identified, the aims of treatment should follow logically from them. A logical structure to use when devising aims/objectives could follow the pattern of: establish the overall aim, identify short- and long-term goals, and then set specific objectives.

Establish aims

Aims are general statements of intent and they provide the basic direction of treatment. The overall aim is usually established in consultation with the team (and constrained by available resources). The following are some fairly typical occupational therapy aims:

- To develop productive occupational role behaviours.
- To discharge home resuming an independent life.
- To undertake graded rehabilitation aiming for discharge to a sheltered environment.
- To improve the quality of life whilst the patient remains in hospital.
- To resettle into part-time employment.
- To learn how to use community resources.

More specific aims can then follow from the general statement, e.g.

- To *improve* a problem area or to increase a skill (e.g. develop conversation skills).
- To *maintain* skill or prevent deterioration (e.g. maintain dressing independence).
- To *minimise* the problem or help adjust to difficulties (e.g. learn alternative methods to communicate).

With the general aims being clearly stated, short- and long-term aims can be realistically constructed. I call these more focused aims 'goals'.

Short- and long-term goals (or aims)

Whilst acknowledging the grey area between 'short-term' and 'long-term' a simple formula can be applied to emphasise their differences. Basically, short-term goals refer to improving immediate *function/skill* or working on the performance components which combine to enable the occupational behaviour (e.g. cognitive function, interpersonal behaviour or task skills). Longer-term goals consider these problem areas in terms of a person's *life roles* (e.g. work, social and domestic aspects, see Table 5.3).

Aims and goals should always be *written* down. Unspecific, mental goals are insufficient. It is too tempting to devise them retrospectively! Once written they can act as something tangible to work towards, and can also be more easily communicated to relevant team members.

Table 5.3 Short- and long-term goals

Short-term goals	Related long-term goals
Improve task performance skills of concentration, sequencing, following instructions, attention to detail, etc.	Check safe level of cooking skills prior to discharge home
Learn relaxation techniques; become more aware of the importance of non-verbal behaviour; demonstrate increased confidence in conversation ability	Practise skills of being interviewed prior to going to an actual job interview

The manner in which these goals are written will vary from unit to unit. Some units might adopt highly regularised procedures, for instance using POMR (problem-orientated medical record) or the SOAP system (problem-based method of recording goals using the headings of subjective, objective, assessment and planning). Also, practitioners vary in whether they write goals for themselves (e.g. *teach* a skill) or from the patient's/client's perspective (e.g. *learn* a skill). The examples in Table 5.3 reflect both methods.

Set specific objectives or outcomes

Objectives as outcome measures

Having established aims and goals, it may be necessary to formulate a step-by-step account of what they entail and how they are to be achieved. Objectives are *precise statements* of intended results or outcomes, and serve as *realistic, measurable targets* for both patient and therapist.

The effective objective includes what is to be achieved, and how, plus the criteria for measuring its achievement. For example, the aim 'to improve the ability to concentrate' can be transformed more precisely into the objective of 'at the end of a month of regular practice, Mr Brown will be able to concentrate for a minimum of 20 minutes on a basic familiar task'. (This might be broken down further, e.g. by the end of the first week, he will be able to concentrate for 10 minute periods.)

THEORY INTO PRACTICE

Setting objectives

Sue becomes acutely anxious when she is required to interact with others. In order to work on these difficulties, she joins the photography group. She has always wanted to pursue photography as a hobby and is keen to develop her skills.

The occupational therapist and Sue negotiate a hierarchy of goals where she is required to interact with others increasingly (and to feel comfortable about it) over the course of 10 sessions (graded exposure).

1. Be a nominal member of the group; work alone taking photographs; interact only with the therapist.
2. Work on an individual activity alongside a group activity.
3. Work with one other person in the group taking photographs outside.
4. Work with the same person in the group room and dark room.
5. Work with another person in the group room and dark room.
6. Join the group when they are being taught a technique; no particular interaction required.
7. Work with others in the group.
8. Join the group in outing to photography museum.

Sue managed goals 1–4 fairly easily by the third session. Her involvement with the photography tasks enabled her to handle the goals for interacting without too much anxiety. On the fourth session, however, Sue had a panic attack prior to going in the dark room with a male member of the group. The planned dark room activity was adapted to accommodate her difficulties. Sue had not anticipated her reaction to the more intimate contact with a man and was able to explore this further in her individual psychotherapy sessions. With extra encouragement and support she achieved the rest of her goals.

Constructing effective objectives

The following points should be remembered when establishing objectives.

1. Goals and objectives should, if possible, be *negotiated* with the patient. At the very least their agreement is needed to ensure the person's co-operation, and hopefully motivation. If an individual does not realise he or she is meant to interact with others to practise the skills, how can we expect him or her to do it? Patients/clients need to know what is expected of them and what they can expect from themselves.
2. Goals and objectives must be *achievable but challenging*. Whilst the overall aim of treatment may require a large leap in the person's functioning (e.g. from being 'ill' to being 'well') it is essential that the person feels he or she can manage the immediate mini-steps. Herein lies the difficulty. There is a fine balance between *stimulation* and too much *pressure*; between underestimating the person's capacity (which results in boredom), and overestimating (which may result in failure and loss of confidence). Because of this, room for failure might need to be built in as 'understandable' or 'acceptable'.
3. Objectives should be *flexible* in adjusting to the person's needs and performance. They therefore need to be regularly re-visited with the patient/client. Ideally, objectives should be made explicit at the beginning of a treatment session. At the end of the session, you then have criteria to evaluate it and future objectives can be modified accordingly.

4. We should recognise that the process of negotiating objectives may, in itself, be *therapeutic*, e.g. trying to establish realistic goals with a person who has an unrealistic self-concept.

Limits of using objectives

On certain occasions it is inappropriate to set objectives. This is particularly the case when working in the more psychodynamic or humanistic traditions. The humanistic approach for example, of letting the client lead (e.g. in non-directive counselling), leaves little room for the therapist to structure future action. In cases like this, aims such as 'gain greater self-awareness' may suffice and, providing the therapist is very clear about the design of treatment (e.g. structure of activity), vague treatment will be avoided.

Objectives are most relevant when modifying behaviour and skills as these can be more readily quantified in terms of outcome measures. The process of learning to type, for instance, can be operationalised into being able to type a certain number of words related to numbers of errors. It is quite a different matter to measure the extent someone is feeling better (though it is possible to have some measures, like the number of minutes engaged in productive activity).

5.3 DESIGNING THE PROGRAMME

We now come to the third stage of planning treatment, i.e. designing the programme. Once the basic aims have been formulated, the more creative side of designing treatment comes into play. Of course, the type of activities offered, and the method of structuring the programme, depends on the particular unit's policy and is clearly constrained by resources available. In general, however, designing a programme will involve manipulating and grading three treatment dimensions in order to maximise therapeutic potential: the *activity*, the *role of therapist* and the *environment*. Let us look in more depth at each of these in turn.

THEORY INTO PRACTICE

Manipulating activity, therapist and environment to improve a person's self-view

Improving a person's negative self-view is not a clear cut problem to work on, as it involves a complicated package of different concerns. As a general guide, the **activity** used in treatment should ideally involve some success experience. Also it could usefully offer opportunities for self-reflection (e.g. a drama mask making two images: 'the outside me' and 'the inside me'). The **therapist** needs to be gentle, supportive and possibly offer the person lots of feedback to facilitate greater self-awareness. A person with an extremely poor self-view will often find it hard to 'take on board' compliments. On the whole offering compliments may be counter-productive. For one thing, they tend to reinforce the message that the therapist is in the business of passing judgements. In terms of the **environment** we need to be cautious not to encourage sick role/dependence on others (e.g. by having too long a hospital stay). Groupwork offers the opportunity to share problems, feedback and support.

Activity

Using activity in treatment

Central to occupational therapy, of course, is our use of activity. As our primary tool we adapt and use activities purposefully to achieve our aims. These aims range from learning and practising skills to expressing and exploring emotions. We have a range of activities at our disposal spanning: individual treatments; large and small groupwork; work, social, domestic aspects; intellectual, physical, hobby interest, etc. The activities themselves are adapted and graded to increase or reduce demands on social, emotional, cognitive, perceptual or physical aspects. Activities are lengthened, shortened, made more complicated, spiced up with competition, rearranged for smaller groups, etc. The following chapter explores this area more fully. The key consideration here is what factors should be taken into account when deciding what activity to use in treatment?

Choosing the best activity

Five factors need to be evaluated:

1. *Aims of treatment* – which activity or activities can best fulfil the aims of treatment, with scope for grading, whilst being appropriate for the patient/client (regarding strengths, difficulties, age, gender and cultural appropriateness)? For example, the structured activities of woodwork or printing are arguably more suitable for improving task performance than an open-ended 'paint what you like' session.
2. *Patient's/client's choice* – which activity is going to be most *meaningful* to the person at both a personal and cultural level? Clearly, motivation to do an activity is increased if it has some meaning for the persona and it is only the individual who can decide this. Whilst the therapist may set some of the parameters, he or she should offer choices to patients/clients respecting their capacity to make their own decisions. As Yerxa points out, 'The meaning of the activity, its choice, and satisfaction in it are determined by the individual patient's needs, interests, and motivations. They should not be determined by the occupational therapist's view of meaning' (1979, p. 29).
3. *Therapist's choice* – sometimes the patient/client is not able to choose which activity he or she would like to do (e.g. when acutely ill). Occupational therapists then choose on the basis of their professional judgement and personal interest. Any therapist needs to have a degree of skill and interest in the chosen

activity – or at the very least a belief in the value of it (particularly important when dealing with patients who lack the necessary motivation).

4. *Practical constraints* – what activities are currently in operation, making the best use of existing resources? For instance, if treatment is to take place in a client's home, our 'activity' might be limited to talking or paper and pencil exercises. Limited funds may constrain opportunities to buy expensive equipment such as computers, kilns, etc. Limited staff resources may prevent certain activities running, e.g. lathework given safety factors. Limited resources can also be a source of inspiration, though, e.g. making 'rubbish collages' which can look very effective!

5. *Balance of overall activity programme* – it is important to consider the shape of the overall programme (e.g. week's timetable) and its total demands on the patient/client. Consider how best to balance the following to suit the individual: new and challenging or reassuring and safe; active or passive; diversional or emotionally charged; restful or stimulating; structure or freedom; staff-directed or patient directed; abstract or concrete. It is a thoughtless institutional practice to ply one's treatment without considering how the patient/client will experience it in the context of a day. I once witnessed the absurd situation of a patient who was required to do cooking all morning with a helper, was assessed at tea time by the occupational therapist in the kitchen and in the evening was pushed into cooking a meal on the ward!

THEORY INTO PRACTICE

Resisting imposing one's own values

As therapists we need to guard against imposing our values/assumptions/stereotypes when we select activities. Take, for example, the cases of Hilda, Karen and Bill:

- Hilda is 72 years old. She is invited to come to the unit's kitchen to cook a meal as part of her domestic assessment prior to discharge. In fact Hilda has always hated cooking. Mostly she buys in frozen TV meals or gets take-aways. The activity that Hilda really wants to do in occupational therapy is have a try on the computer. She has always wanted to have a go but has felt shy about asking!
- Karen, aged 20, is encouraged to help a group of patients put up Christmas decorations. At first she is reluctant but after much persuasion she makes some streamers. Later the occupational therapist found out that Karen got into trouble with her parents who are Jehovah's Witnesses and do not support celebrating Christmas in this way.
- Bill, aged 65, watches television all day. The therapist feels it would be beneficial for Bill to be engaged in something 'more productive' and suggests a range of community activities. Bill is not interested and disengages from treatment.

Role of therapist

Therapist use of self as a treatment tool

A much-used, yet often unexplored aim of treatment is to 'establish rapport'. What exactly do we mean? It seems to be a phrase we use to acknowledge the fundamental importance of the relationship between patient/client and therapist. Often, the quality of our relationship is the significant factor in the progress of treatment. If a patient does not trust us, he or she is unlikely to follow our recommendations. Sometimes patients/clients will believe in us first rather than believing in the treatment.

As part of our relationship we adapt our approach and role. We need to consider how best to encourage and motivate our patients/clients, and make them feel safe. Does the individual respond best to our manner when we are gentle?; forceful?; humorous?; directive? What role should we play? Consider the following range of possibilities: teacher, advice-giver, meeter of needs, model of normality, psychotherapist, behaviour-reinforcer, equipment supplier, facilitator, etc. Often, we adapt and modify our role as treatment progresses. In rehabilitation, for example, we grade our expectations by increasing the amount of autonomy and independence we give our patients/clients. We gradually reduce our support and direction, handing over responsibility. Arguably the most potent element of treatment is our 'conscious use of self' in a therapeutic manner, i.e. therapists use themselves as *a treatment tool*.

THEORY INTO PRACTICE

Responding and being sensitive to individuals' needs

Jennifer says she feels fat, ugly and horrible. She is in fact attractive and has much to offer. Her therapist thinks through how she should handle this: 'I don't think Jennifer wants reassurance here. She may find it useful to hear me state the reality as I see it. Yet I suspect she isn't going to be able to take any compliments on board. Anyway if I entered into evaluation (however positive) I would give off messages that I am judging her. Her perception is what is important. So my approach will be to acknowledge her poor self-image and focus on trying to change her negative thinking.'

Rowena says she feels dowdy and horrible after 2 weeks in hospital. Her therapist decides a practical response is needed. She confirms that it is the hospital stay that is bringing Rowena down. They then discuss what might counteract the effects. Rowena settles on spending an afternoon at her hairdresser's when she goes home at the weekend. In the meantime she takes up the therapist's suggestion of putting on some make-up.

Deciding what approach

The decision of what approach and role we take on can be determined by a range of factors.

First and foremost, we need to *respond sensitively* to the individual's needs. One person might enjoy being jollied along, whilst another needs a quieter, gentler approach. Often the most skilled therapists are skilled because they seem to have the ability to 'strike the right note' and respond in a way that respects anothers' way of operating.

Secondly, the *situation and activity* is clearly a determinant of our approach. We are likely to be more directive if we need to manage a large group of patients, as opposed to one-to-one situations. Different activities also require different role-taking, such as being a 'teacher' when introducing a new task. The respective personalities involved also need considering. For example, a manner that works for one therapist could fail with another simply because it comes across as artificial (a lesson here from counselling where 'genuineness' is seen as a core quality).

Next, the *team approach* often guides our methods, such as when the team decides a patient needs consistent handling or assigns a key worker to respond in a certain way (e.g. be confrontative). Our approach also has to mesh with colleagues with whom we may be working (i.e. co-therapists complementing each other). Here, for example, one of the team may take a directive role controlling the group, while the other is supportive of individuals. In the times when staff shortages pre-empt such careful structuring, extra efforts should be made to guide nurses, students and helpers when they join in therapy sessions, regarding how they could best contribute in an unfamiliar situation.

Finally, the *theoretical framework* we are working within is, of course, a big influence. At a broad level our professional philosophy suggests we should be client centred and foster an egalitarian relationship that invites participation. More specifically, our treatment approach can guide our responses. For instance, in the humanistic tradition we would incline towards being non-directive and accepting to encourage self-expression. As a behaviourist we might be more directive in the way we reinforce behaviour and offer a structure for the patient.

THEORY INTO PRACTICE

Some guidelines for approaching different people

An anxious person
Genuine reassurance given in a quiet, calm manner should be the main strategy used. Also valuable is our use of any 'relaxing' absorbing (thus diverting) activity, if the person can be persuaded to join in. The key decision to make is whether or not he or she will benefit most from an undemanding or structured environment – the person may appreciate being free to settle when ready, or may need the security of outside direction where the onus for any decision-making is removed.

A suspicious/deluded person

Two main 'rules' apply here: (a) try to keep conversation (and activity) on a concrete, straightforward plane, and (b) avoid getting locked into circular discussions and trying to reason the person out of his or her beliefs. An initial clear explanation about the situation is important (e.g. 'The way I see it is ...'), but it is unlikely to help to keep repeating your view. Diversionary tactics may work, such as 'before we talk more about that' can you try to concentrate on this activity for a few minutes?' Another possible strategy is to empathise with what is 'real', e.g. not responding to the person's fear of 'outer space electricity', but responding to their fear.

A potentially suicidal person

The highly emotive issue of potential suicide can only be handled if we take any threats seriously and try to minimise our own value judgements (and advice as to why he or she should live). When faced with a person expressing a wish to die, our best role is to listen and allow him or her to express the tensions which have lead to this point. Any suicidal patient/client should be carefully monitored by the team, with general precautions (e.g. not leaving the patient alone, removing scissors) being taken as necessary. We should not have an actively suicidal person in activity groups unless we have adequate staff resources to give one-to-one attention if necessary.

A confused, disorientated person

Reassurance, routine and structure are the important elements here. The person's daily programme and environment should be well-organised and consistent. Devices such as written timetables and clear signposts are helpful, especially when combined with the human touch, where the therapist gently and clearly repeats basic information. As with any management strategy, it is most successful when applied consistently by the team.

A person whose behaviour is uncontrolled/hyperactive

There are many strategies which might be tried, according to what the individual responds to best. Whilst ignoring the behaviour may help, the reverse can also be true (e.g. giving a little extra attention or reassuring physical contact may prevent the behaviour escalating). In any case, the therapist should give the individuals some feedback on what is difficult about the behaviour and allow them the opportunity to take responsibility for controlling themselves. When the behaviour is so disturbed it disrupts the rest of a group, the individual may need to be temporarily excluded (a one-to-one activity may be more appropriate at this stage anyway). Activities requiring aggressive/gross motions may help to release some tensions, but often they also increase arousal, so should be used carefully.

An aggressive person

Possibly the most difficult aspect of coping with verbal or physical aggression is our own reactions to violence and controlling them. In most circumstances the therapist needs to set and maintain clear, consistent limits of what is acceptable, and enforce them when necessary (telling the patient to leave the group). If there is no physical danger to anyone at stake (e.g. verbal abuse), the situation should be handled in a calm, matter-of-fact way designed to diffuse rather than provoke anger. If physical violence occurs, it needs to be dealt with immediately, so be clear about your unit's policy/procedures. Whilst we must try to ensure the safety of all patients/clients, we also have a right to keep ourselves free from physical harm. The team is an important support when any of us suffer from the understandable anxieties that occur, following a violent incident.

Environment

In therapy the environment consists of *the human element* of the people around and their attitudes, and the *non-human* aspects of the physical surroundings. These are manipulated in many subtle ways to achieve a range of goals. As Kielhofner notes, 'The only tool which therapists have at their disposal is to change the relevant environment to support or precipitate change' (1995, p. 261).

First, the occupational therapy area needs to fit its purpose. Often it acts as an area where patients/clients are expected to take on active and different roles, particularly if they have taken passive or sick roles elsewhere. If required, the environment also needs to be suited to the learning of new skills, which necessarily applies both to physical equipment and emotional support. Thus we manipulate our environment in terms of providing varied and selected stimulation to maximise learning and effective functioning. Here we darken rooms for relaxation, simulate industrial therapy workshops, provide free expression, graffiti walls and so on. We also carefully balance quiet spaces with active, more noisy sections. The options are endless and depend much on the needs of the patient/client group as well as available resources – the key is that we recognise its importance.

Secondly, a significant part of the environment is **people**. The influence of the therapist's role had already been discussed. Beyond this, the influence of other people can be crucial (e.g. with groupwork). Choice of group size is itself important (six to eight patients, or less if they are disturbed, is the usual small group number) and is often dependent on an assessment of how mutually supportive the group members are likely to be and on their developmental levels.

Thirdly, the other human, though less tangible, aspect is the **atmosphere and attitudes** of people around. What 'feel' does the department have? Caring? Busy? Accepting? Do patients feel encouraged? If the answers are in the negative, is there anything that can be done to change the 'feel' in more positive directions?

Fourthly, the **physical environment** in terms of type of room, comfort, arrangements of seating and positioning, layout of equipment, etc. are all very relevant aspects. Slight modifications in any of these can have dramatic effects on people's performance and attitudes (e.g. using floor cushions rather than chairs to promote an informal, relaxed atmosphere; sitting a group around in a circle to promote interaction; or putting up dividers to make a space feel more private).

Lastly, the **therapeutic environment** is never static. The treatment process involves continually exploiting, modifying and adapting the environment. It is the process of grading the environment (namely adding more stimulation, pressure, stress) which makes the treatment effective. Thus patients/clients move from individual to group sessions; from hospital to community-based sessions; from structured to unstructured environments.

THEORY INTO PRACTICE

Grading the environment

Neeta, aged 25, suffers from extreme social anxieties which paralyse her whenever she is in the same room as other people. On a one-to-one level, Neeta is able to function well, being bright and articulate. As part of the wider treatment, the therapist and Neeta negotiate a systematic desensitisation programme where she is exposed to increasing levels of social contact in the environment.

Level 1 Work one-to-one with therapist in a large workroom but away from others behind a screen.
Level 2 Screen partially removed so Neeta catches glimpses of others.
Level 3 Screen removed but therapist acts as a protective screen.
Level 4 Neeta and therapist work in the open (other people are around doing their own activities but keep away).
Level 5 One other person (of Neeta's choice) joins the activity session.
Level 6 Size of group increased.

Neeta achieved all levels within 3 weeks. Whilst the programme looks as though it would take a long time, Neeta progressed swiftly as she felt safe enough to take some risks.

SUMMARY

The stages of planning treatment can be summarised as shown in Figure 5.2.

5.4 CASE ILLUSTRATIONS

Case illustration 5.1: 'Thomas'

Thomas, aged 35, has a long-standing history of unstable epilepsy and a tendency towards being passive and dependent in his behaviour. He was admitted to an acute unit to stabilise his medication. On initial assessment the occupational therapist learned he lived in a flat with his parents and spent most of his time watching television. When he was feeling better, he helped around the house more.

The team recognised Thomas was likely to be discharged in a couple of weeks, so there was a limit to how much treatment could be accomplished, but they were concerned about what was likely to happen on his discharge. Based on his previous pattern of being erratic about taking his medication, it seemed likely he would be readmitted within a few months. It was agreed that the occupational

Organise information
(1) Process all assessment information
(2) Identify problems in functional terms
(3) Identify strengths to build on
(4) Select priority problem(s)

Establish aims and goals
(1) Establish overall aim
(2) Identify short- and long-term aims or goals
(3) Set specific objectives where relevant

Design the programme, arranging:

(1) *Activity* – the choice of which activity and how demanding to make it depends on treatment aims, patient's/client's preference, therapist's selection, practical constraints and overall programme balance. Where possible, we should try to be client-centred and only use activities which the individual finds meaningful. Consider how to grade the activity in order to achieve treatment aims (e.g. increase complexity of task to facilitate higher learning of problem-solving skill).

(2) *Role of therapist* – therapist's role includes the general approach to a patient or client, specific ways of handling behaviour and the use of self/relationship as a therapeutic tool. It depends on the theoretical framework, situation, personalities involved, etc. Consider how to grade your role in order to achieve the desired aim (e.g. become less directive and reduce support to encourage greater independence to the patient or client).

(3) *Environment* – environment includes people involved and their attitudes and physical structures. Consider how to set up the environment in order to achieve your aim (e.g. reduce amount of tools available for use to encourage sharing between people).

Figure 5.2 Summary of how to plan treatment.

therapist would attempt to function more as a bridge between the hospital and community.

The occupational therapist decided the most useful intervention would be to try to help Thomas develop some new productive activity which he would be able to continue once discharged. The therapist reasoned that having a new role or interest would not only give Thomas more drive/motivation, it would offer a way of structuring his day (which would have a positive spin-off for maintaining his mental health).

The first step of treatment then was to search for a meaningful occupation. Thomas was unresponsive when she tried to interview him. She returned to the occupational therapy records from his previous admissions. The therapist discovered Thomas had always loved plants/nature and often could be found wandering around the local parks and gardens. Also, he had functioned well in previous occupational therapy gardening groups, though this had not been taken further.

The therapist returned to Thomas and asked if he would like to come back to do some gardening. For the first time in his admission, he showed a spark of interest. They agreed a *short-term* aim that he would come down to the department daily to re-learn and practice his gardening skills (e.g. potting plants, taking cuttings, etc.). For the *long term*, the therapist hoped he would become sufficiently engaged to take on the responsibility to create a patio garden at home.

Thomas spent 2 weeks attending to the unit's plants. Towards the end of his admission, he went with the therapist to a garden centre to plan and plant up a new tub of flowers for the unit's entrance. Thomas became interested in the suggestion of a patio garden and he used his remaining days in the hospital to plan this. On his discharge, the therapist arranged she would visit him at three-weekly intervals, with the aim of continuing to encourage the new hobby and to monitor his use of medication.

Grading
- *Activity* – graded gardening: first practising skills on pot plants in the department; then visiting the garden centre and doing some long-term planning; finally designing and maintaining own patio garden.
- *Role* – initially therapist more directive, e.g. giving instruction; later encouraging Thomas to make his own decisions and supporting him to be independent
- *Environment* – hospital; then some community involvement; then home-based support

Case illustration 5.2: Leisure group

A twice weekly leisure group was developed for 10 elderly clients being treated in a day unit. In the first session, with the therapists help, the clients decided on a regular music appreciation slot amongst other activities. The therapist made the following treatment plan.

Ideas for different activities
1. Each member bring in a special piece of music and share reminiscences.
2. Briefly discuss the life and times of the composer, band leader, etc.
3. Respond to a new piece of music and share reactions with other group members.

Aims of treatment
1. Reactivate an interest in music and encourage its use as a hobby.
2. Encourage group interaction and relationship building.
3. Enable personal reminiscences and expression of feelings.

Grading
- *Activity* – Initially less threatening emphasis on hobby interest moving on to more personal and interpersonal elements.
- *Role* – Initially therapist more involved, actively prompting, etc. Later try to hand over decision making, etc., to group.
- *Environment* – Circle of comfortable chairs; as relationships develop introduce more intimacy (e.g. dancing).

THEORY INTO PRACTICE

How to use activity, therapist role and environment to motivate

Perhaps the most common problem confronting us in the mental health field is when patients/clients lack motivation to engage in treatment. If we find a patient/client does not want to join the occupational therapy activity, then our first task is to disentangle what is causing the lack of motivation.

Activity
Invariably, motivation will be increased if the patient/client can identify with the purpose and value of treatment. It is our job to clarify how and why treatment might be relevant and to ensure the activities are meaningful. Ideally the patient/client should be actively involved in planning his or her own treatment. This not only engages them in treatment, it ensures they take some responsibility for future progress.

Approach
Can the person's reluctance to attend occupational therapy be put down to uncertainty, anxiety or confusion about the purpose of treatment? In this case, careful explanation and preparation is needed where the individual has time to air any concerns and questions. All too often we forget how difficult it can be to go to a new place and meet new people. We can also forget how threatening treatment can be.

Environment
Does the person lack drive as a product of his or her illness, institutionalisation or medication? If this is the case, care needs to be taken to make the treatment environment (and activity) reasonably stimulating, rewarding and enjoyable for the individual. In addition, it might be possible to use other patients/clients as a model or as a source of information about their experiences of occupational therapy.

CONCLUSION

This chapter has laid out the stages of the treatment planning process, exploring the way therapists reason and the criteria they bring to bear in making clinical decisions. The main points are summarised in Figure 5.2.

Before leaving the subject I would like to reiterate a note of balance. I have presented the treatment process as involving three clear cut stages. In practice these are not clear cut. Mostly, the process does not occur in a set sequence – often aims/goals are revisited and modified. Sometimes treatment starts by doing an activity and the planning occurs subsequently. As Mattingly and Fleming (1994) strongly argue, simply focusing on the occupational therapy process does not reflect the complexity and flexibility of the way therapists actually think and act. Also, 'change' in our patients/clients is rarely orderly. As Kielhofner puts it 'change involves periods of stability and instability, dramatic transformation and uneven progression' (1995, p. 259). Treatment needs to be flexible and adapt to such evolution.

That said, in the end, trying to be clear and systematic in the treatment planning will enable treatment to be both coherent and effective. If therapists cannot be clear about the treatment process, what chance does the patient/client have of understanding it, let alone carrying it out?

Discussion questions

1. What are the differences between aims and objectives? Give examples, recognising the difference between therapist-centred and patient-centred aims.
2. The aim 'establish rapport' is unhelpful and too simplistic. Discuss.
3. What aspects of treatment can be manipulated and graded, and how?
4. What should we do if a patient refuses to, or is unable to, participate in treatment planning?
5. It could be argued that an occupational therapists' time is better spent treating patients/clients where a successful outcome is likely, rather than working with people with long-standing intractable problems. What would you say in response to this?
6. Should therapists approach (i.e. handle, relate to) patients/clients strategically as opposed to being natural and spontaneous?

Occupation and activity in treatment

6

Activity is the core of occupational therapy. Our concept of activity operates at two levels. First, we focus on how illness/problems affect a person's daily life *occupations*. Secondly, we use *activities* in the treatment process.

Our belief in the centrality of occupations and the healing power of activities has largely defined our profession over the years. Early pioneers emphasised how the health of individuals could be influenced by purposeful activities, by 'the use of muscles and mind together in games', exercise and handicraft, as well as in work (Hopkins, 1983, p. 3). However, what does activity offer and why do we use it? Why do occupational therapists put so much store in 'doing' being active and involved? When we say activity is purposeful and therapeutic what do we mean?

This chapter seeks to explore the role of occupations in our society and to demonstrate ways in which the purposeful use of activity is therapeutic. First, I will start by analysing the social context of occupations and activity. Then I will explore the therapeutic value of activities used in occupational therapy. A final section will present several case illustrations of how activities are applied in practice.

Before exploring these questions, however, let us be clear about the use of terms occupation and activity.* My way of distinguishing between these is to consider **occupations** as a person's purposeful daily life roles in the areas of *work, leisure and self-care*. To carry out these roles a person performs numerous activities (e.g. a secretary types, takes short-hand). It is these *daily activities* (sometimes referred to as 'purposeful activities') which we can employ in occupational therapy, along with *other therapeutic activities*. Daily living activities include activities related to work, leisure and self-care, for instance we may encourage a secretary to prac-tise her typing or a housewife to go shopping. Therapeutic activities tend only to

---

* Controversy continues to surround these concepts. I would recommend studying the Mocellin's (1995, 1996) critique of the use of occupation as a core concept for occupational therapy. For a deeper explorations of the ideas underlying the use of occupation and activity I would recommend: (a) the American Occupational Therapy Association (1995) Position paper on occupation and (b) the discussion on 'adjunctive' versus 'enabling' activities in Predretti (1996).

take place in a treatment context (e.g. groupwork, art therapy and anxiety management). See Figure 6.1.

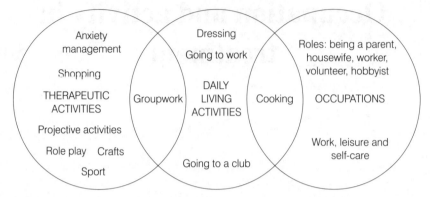

Figure 6.1 Therapeutic versus daily living activities and occupations.

Whilst we can distinguish between occupations, daily living activities and therapeutic activities, the categories also overlap. For instance, clerical work tasks could be seen as daily living activities for a person whose occupation is a secretary and used as part of a work rehabilitation programme. Those same tasks could be used therapeutically to improve another person's (who is not a secretary) task performance skills. As another example, cooking could be used both to assess domestic independence skills (daily living activity) and as a nurturing, gratifying activity (therapeutic activity). The key point is how the activity is *applied*. For a deeper, comprehensive analysis of these concepts I recommend chapter 5 in Hagedorn (1995).

6.1 THE SOCIAL CONTEXT OF ACTIVITY

Kielhofner defines human occupation as, 'doing culturally meaningful work, play or daily living tasks in the stream of time and in the contexts of one's physical and social world' (1995, p. 3). In other words, any occupation or activity needs to be understood as arising in a social and cultural context. This notion is such an important one for occupational therapists I think it is beneficial to probe it further. The 'social' can be seen to play a role at three levels. Firstly, occupations have a *social basis*. Secondly, all activities are *socially constructed*. Thirdly, *culture* plays a significant role in giving meaning to activities. Each of these points will be discussed below.

Social basis of occupations

Occupations have a social basis because they involve *social roles* (at work, at home, at leisure). Kielhofner is more explicit and describes occupations as comprising of three general areas of behaviour: play, daily living tasks and work. Play, the earliest occurring occupational behaviour, includes all forms of exploring, pretending, gaming and creating. Daily living tasks include self-care activities and routine domestic tasks. Work refers to both paid and unpaid functions carried out as an employee, student parent, serious hobbyist, etc.

Occupations can also be understood as having a social basis as the very definition of what constitutes work and play are a product of *society's norms and ideas*. Ideologies in our society carry images of what are appropriate occupations for different groups of people. For example, in our culture, elderly people are supposed to retire from paid work and children are supposed to play. In other cultures, elders are the community leaders and children are required to work. In our culture, it is accepted that both men and women seek employment. In other cultures men may be expected to be the bread winner whilst the women stay at home.

A final way that occupations have a social basis is that the meanings individuals attach to their occupations may well depend on their *social circumstances*. For instance, an unemployed person may regard their degree studies with the Open University as 'work', whilst someone who is in paid employment may choose to do a degree for leisure! One individual may paint for pleasure, but this definition could change if he or she was offered a commission.

Social construction of activity

People are occupational beings. We go through life being active. We adopt different roles and carry out different activities at different points in our life span. Whilst we can view this as a 'natural' process, part of evolution, I would argue that society not only plays a crucial role in constructing our occupations but also shapes what and how activities are performed. Activities are also socially constructed as we learn how to do them through our social relationships and interactions.

Think of any situation where a person is involved in activity. Imagine a girl playing with a doll, for instance. Now develop the scene. Say she is playing on the floor in front of her parents. It is her birthday, she has just received this doll, her parents are smiling benignly, taking pleasure in her pleasure. The girl starts to play a bit roughly with the doll and is gently reprimanded saying she must 'take care of the pretty baby doll!'.

In this example, we can see the social context is relevant in two ways: at the macro level concerning society's expectations and at the micro level of social interactions. At the *macro-social* level, we could make several comments about how society defines what is appropriate children's activity (i.e. play), or what is an appropriate toy in our culture (e.g. doll). Society even lays down how we do the activity (for instance using a doll symbolically like a baby). Our Western culture is also relevant in this story as the way we celebrate birthdays by giving a person presents is a culturally specific practice. At a *micro-social* level, we can see that the girl's behaviour is being influenced by her parents – their choice of gift and expectations to do with it, their smiles, their reprimands. Their (and other peoples') expectations and responses will similarly shape how the girl performs other activities and her attitudes to them.

The role of culture

The necessity for occupational therapists to recognise the importance of culture regarding both occupations and activities is exemplified when we look at the role of work and leisure in our society and when we consider different cultural practices.

Role of work and leisure

The role of (paid) work in contemporary UK society has changed dramatically in the last decades. The type of work available has changed – both in terms of de-skilling and re-skilling as a result of the expansion of technology and automation. Perhaps the most dramatic changes have been the rise in unemployment which has resulted in the expansion of leisure and variations in types of work (such as part-time work, job share and voluntary work).

Not surprisingly this has had a major impact on occupational therapy. For one thing, much greater emphasis is placed on leisure and general time management rather than work rehabilitation (particularly in view of the stigma of mental illness and how that impacts on ex-patients not being given job opportunities).

We also need to guard against our own assumptions that patients/clients should have, or need, a work role. We would do well to avoid trying to impose our own view about what being 'productive' entails as each individual will differ. Take for example a patient who is being 'resettled' into the community. If a person's number one leisure activity is to hang around the shopping mall, shouldn't this be seen as productive in his or her terms?

The key point here is to recognise how definitions of work and leisure vary according to different cultures. It is important to look at what work/leisure means to an individual and how it is experienced. For this reason, Primeau (1996) warns us about thinking in terms of the false dichotomy of work and leisure.

Different cultural practices and values

The significance of not imposing our own values is even more sharply illustrated when we consider cross-cultural practices about how activities should be performed. Imaging the following situation. You are doing a kitchen assessment observing how a man makes tea. He proceeds to put tea leaves into the kettle on the hob. So you step in to assist. You (reasonably) deduce he is confused and possibly his visual perception/object recognition is somewhat impaired. This is in fact a true story and it happened to a friend of mine. What the occupational therapist did not realise was that my friend had come from an African village where they boil tea in a kettle with milk and sugar. Had the therapist given my friend the electric kettle, he would have made it the Western way!

As another example, consider the client who cut up slices of her birthday cake with her fingers. Initially staff were concerned to see this display of 'bad manners'. They later learned the client was an orthodox Jew who would have felt unable to eat the cake if a hospital kitchen knife (which was not Kosher) had been used.

THEORY INTO PRACTICE

Therapists should avoid imposing their own cultural values

One example of a situation where a therapist unthinkingly imposed her own values occurred on a home visit with a Bangladeshi woman. She had been referred as she was suffering tearfulness and anxiety. On interview the therapist discovered her client did not have any 'leisure' occupations because she spent several hours everyday cooking elaborate meals for her large family. The woman also cared for two children under the age of 5 and an ageing infirm uncle. The occupational therapist diagnosed stress and tried to encourage the woman to take some time off, e.g. using convenience meals or getting her husband to cook. The point the therapist missed, however, was that the woman's caring activities were both valued and expected, and she enjoyed doing them! Further the shame/distress the woman would feel at not carrying out her 'role' properly could have been far more damaging than any benefit from having more leisure time.

The examples above illustrate the need for us to be aware that peoples' attitudes and meanings about daily activities and how they should be performed are culturally embedded. We could go even further and recognise how our therapy practice and our values are, themselves, culturally shaped. For example, take our concept of 'promoting independence' – a major value of occupational therapy. Independence is as, Kinebanian and Stomph (1992) remind us, a 'Western, white, middle-class value. It is associated with making one's own decisions, having freedom of choice, knowing what one wants to achieve in life, and accepting personal responsibility'. They go on to describe how in many non-western societies, values such as honouring the family and accepting other peoples' decisions are far more important than independence. As they say, 'dependency is a respectable choice' (1992, p. 752).

If our interventions are to have a chance at being effective, we need to recognise the cultural biases and assumptions underpinning our professional practice.

6.2 THE THERAPEUTIC VALUE OF ACTIVITY

This section aims to explore the therapeutic value of activities by approaching activities in three ways. First, the intrinsic value of activities will be identified.

Then the range and value of activities used in occupational therapy will be explored. The final section will describe how occupational therapists analyse activities in order to make them therapeutic.

Intrinsic value of activity

Activity is fundamental to human existence in that we have an innate, spontaneous tendency to be active and to explore our world. We also need to be active in order to survive and have a degree of quality of life. Activities – both the process of doing them and their end-product – have value at many different levels, and we can see this applied both to ourselves and to therapy (see Figure 6.2).

1. We use activity as a *learning tool* to help us explore ourselves, others and the environment. Along with learning we gain awareness of our own capacity, *a sense of competence*, effectiveness, esteem and mastery (Mocellin, 1995). A child's use of activity, in the form of play, clearly illustrates how one can use it to practise/learn skills and to test out knowledge and perceptions.
2. Activity also *activates us*. It motivates and energises us at a physical and mental level, stimulating the senses. Consider the times you have felt lethargic and sluggish, but after some exercise have felt revitalised.
3. The process of engaging in activity can be a form of play and has *social value*. It can be both pleasurable and diversional. At the very least it is something to do; at best we can have fun, be sociable and relate to others.
4. Activity can be a vehicle *to express and explore feelings*. For example, writing a diary has a projective function in that it can release tensions and be cathartic.
5. Activity is *productive*. Both the process of doing and the end-product can be gratifying. Being purposeful and creative meets our esteem needs plus carries tangible rewards (such as the end-product or monetary value, etc.).

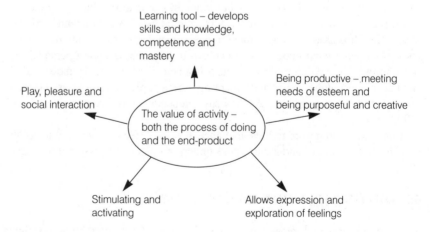

Figure 6.2 Value of activity.

Behind any notion of the value of activity is an acknowledgement that activity has the potential to meet 'needs' at every level. This can be illustrated by using Maslow's (1954) 'hierarchy of needs' as a reference. Cooking, for example, offers opportunities to satisfy: physiological needs, if a person is hungry; esteem needs, if he or she receives praise; mastery needs, as the individual learns new skills; and self-actualisation needs, if he or she simply enjoys cooking. Groupwork, as another example, can offer an individual the opportunity to have their love and belonging needs met when they are accepted by the group, as well as esteem needs met, if they are recognised as having an important contribution to make.

Thus occupational therapists believe in activity for all its inherent values. We also, however, place emphasis on activities being *structured*, *adapted* and *graded* purposefully within treatment. Thus, we analyse activities in order to understand their component parts and inherent demands. Then we carefully apply the activity to suit an individual or group in order to enhance their functioning. Generally occupational therapists modify, and therapeutically use, activities with five main aims in mind.

- *To assess* a person's occupational performance and measure any progress in the future.
- To improve specific *areas of deficit*, e.g. cognitive skills being improved with extra training using quizzes and work tasks.
- To *raise self-esteem* of the person by facilitating awareness about his or her capacities/potential and developing confidence as a result of achievement.
- To provide an enjoyable, *social outlet* through activities.
- To help people *acquire new skills*, e.g. to help the patient cope better in the present, as seen in relaxation, or for the future, such as when we suggest a new hobby.

Occupational therapy activities

There are a vast number of activities at the disposal of occupational therapists, for theoretically, we can use any activity that is legal! Our choice is constrained, of course, by what the patients/clients want to do themselves, the aims of our treatment and the resources available to us (see section on 'choosing the best activity' in Chapter 5). The selection of appropriate and meaningful activities is not easy. Then, care needs to be taken to *apply* the activity therapeutically (e.g. appropriately analysing and then grading it). In other words we do not just use any old activity. Rather we analyse a wide range of possible activities and learn to apply a few, purposefully and in a skillful manner, for the benefit of our patients/clients.

Given the above points there are a number of activities which seem to turn up regularly in our repertoire, within occupational therapy programmes (hospital or day units). Some of these will be briefly described and evaluated, to give a flavour of their aims and therapeutic use.

Occupational therapy activities are commonly described in terms of their content as pertaining to work, social, domestic or personal aspects of daily life (i.e.

self-care, productivity and leisure). It is perhaps equally useful to describe the range of activities in terms of their basic *aims and processes*. In exploring this latter notion we can view activities along a spectrum,* moving from task activities where emphasis is placed on teaching skills to psychotherapy activities which aim to explore feelings (Figure 6.3). A range of social and communication activities fall somewhere between task and psychotherapy activities. These divisions are not rigid as:

1. Most activities can be adapted to fit into one or other category depending on the desired aim. Art, for example, can be equally used as a work task or projectively.
2. Any one activity can simultaneously fit into several levels, e.g. a pottery work group may also be a social gathering.
3. Each individual will respond differently to an activity. Embroidery may be a relaxing social activity for a person skilled in it, but a daunting challenge for the uninitiated.

The following four sections examine these activity groupings in more detail. The descriptions offered are necessarily brief, but serve as examples showing the richness and variety of occupational therapy activities. Throughout these sections, references for research relating to how specific activities can be applied therapeutically are indicated. Research substantiating our practice (a necessary development in the context of evidence based practice and the demands to measure outcomes) is still in its infancy but the pool of evidence is growing.

Task activities

Task activities aim to improve our daily living, work or task performance skills. They can be run at every level, from trying to improve concentration in a craft group to work simulation and training.

Cookery

Cooking is a commonly used occupational therapy activity, mainly because it can be so easily graded whilst being almost universally practical. It offers opportunities for people to develop task performance skills (e.g. following instructions, problem solving), and can also be applied to later stages of treatment when patients are practising their domestic role skills (e.g. home management units using cookery as part of wider domestic rehabilitation). Cooking seems to be enjoyed by people of all age groups and abilities, not least because of enjoyable end-products.

   Research by Kremer, Nelson and Duncombe (1984) confirms these points (though their study was small scale and would benefit from being replicated). They investigated the degree of meaning different activities held for chronic psychiatric patients. They randomly assigned 22 patients to three groups: cooking,

---

* Borg and Bruce (1991) offer a similar continuum classification in their separation of psychotherapy groups, therapeutic activity groups and traditional task groups.

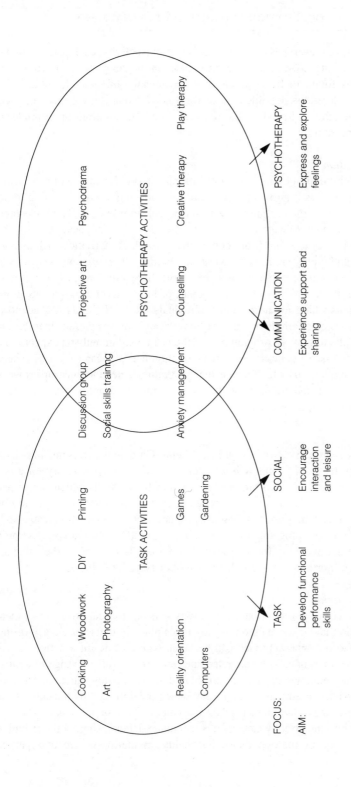

Figure 6.3 Spectrum of occupational therapy activities (after Finlay, 1997).

craft and sensory awareness groups. After the group activity, each patient rated its affective meaning. Results showed differences in meaning for each activity and cooking was found to be significantly more meaningful than the others. The authors considered the possible reasons for this were that it is a concrete activity with a consumable end-product; it offers oral stimulation; it is age appropriate and culturally meaningful.

Work simulation

Work rehabilitation in today's economic climate is problematic, and is now usually geared towards improving work skills and offering a work role (e.g. doing DIY in the home), rather than towards vocational resettlement. The widespread use of sheltered factory workshops offering assembly lines for packaging, etc., has diminished in recent years. More commonly these days, activities such as computer work and typing are used for work simulation. Otherwise, any task activity, for instance woodwork, can be used for 'work hardening' or to develop work skills. Often these activities are used as part of longer term programmes in day centres or units which aim to maintain individuals' skills. Nichol (1984) acknowledges the absence of employment opportunities and advises therapists to be cautious when planning work programmes as they can instil unrealistic expectations. Oxley (1995) discusses how a work rehabilitation needs to cater for a wide spectrum of people's needs which means that programmes need to encompass works skills assessment and training, sheltered or supported employment, and for a minority, preparation for open employment.

Gardening

Horticulture is attractive to many patients/clients. Gardening offers much, as it can be graded from simple window box watering to taking responsibility for a vegetable plot. It provides opportunities to learn new hobby skills which can be realistically applied, for example, on discharge, as well as opportunities to nurture something which can grow and tangibly produce rewards. Gardening can also be beneficial for developing cognitive function where individuals can practise problem solving and planning for the future. For a good description of the value and application of horticulture, see Gibson (1996) or Hagedorn (1996).

Reality orientation

The specific use of reality orientation activity sessions to treat problems of memory, confusion and disorientation usually takes place in units for elderly people. Here a classroom-type approach can be taken where basic information (e.g. of day, date, weather, names) is reiterated and reinforced, whilst a range of appropriate activities, e.g. memory games, are geared to maximising function. The most successful reality orientation remains that which is reinforced by the entire team, and recognises the individual's needs and dignity (a 24-hour approach). The body of research into the effectiveness of this technique is increasing, with the bulk of evidence supporting the hypothesis that reality orientation is effective, particularly when used by the team to combat confusion. Evidence concerning the value of memory activities is mixed and some therapists argue reality orientation can be patronising, or even, at times, unkind (for instance when reminding people about a bereavement). Care must be taken to apply it humanely and meaningfully (e.g. gearing activities towards social interaction rather than simply reinforcing the date and time). For more in-depth discussions on research and applications, see Holden and Woods (1988).

THEORY INTO PRACTICE

Example activity evaluation: *Pottery*

Value
1. Improves task performance skills, e.g. concentration, following instructions, attention to detail.
2. Easily graded for those with different skill levels, to ensure successful end-product.
3. Outlet for creativity and self-expression.
4. Offers tactile/sensory experience.
5. Hobby interest and leisure pursuit (e.g. night classes).
6. Used in graded programmes, e.g. for tolerance to dirt.

Ways of adapting
1. Length of process and patient involvement, e.g. from wedging to firing, or just making a pot.
2. Activity itself – thumb pots, coil pots, slab pots, decorative tiles, wheel, sculpture, group collage such as a village scene, etc.
3. Types of equipment – clay, 'Playdoh', plasticine, flour and water, or use of different tools and machinery.

Considerations
1. Messiness, e.g. for some it can be distressing.
2. Ensuring success versus not protecting patient from failure (make this decision for each individual).
3. Resources – can be expensive, a separate area may be required, a skilled technician may be useful to make good, mistakes and offer high-level teaching/ideas.
4. Length of time for whole process, e.g. some people need immediate results and may find the wait for the glazed product difficult.

Social activities

The wide spectrum of social activities are primarily aimed at promoting interaction, enjoyment and leisure interests. For a more in-depth look at leisure, see Ravetz (1996).

Crafts
The range of crafts, from traditional activities such as basketry to more recently

introduced activities such as photography, offer much for every age group and ability level. A group of people sitting in a circle whilst engaged in a craft is a common sight in many day units. These activities are both useful for task skills and provide a focal point for social interaction. The most successful craft departments seem to be those where clear aims are pursued and products are attractively displayed or sold (rather than being thrown away or re-used).

The research base validating the use of activities/crafts is growing. McDermott (1988) considered the effect of three types of group treatments (using pottery/art group; activity-based discussion group; verbal group without activity). She found that the craft activities produced more positive socio-emotional communications (compliments, expressed satisfaction, joking), more interactions between members and fewer uninvolved members, than with the more verbal groups. Klyczek and Mann (1986) compared two different treatment programmes one offering more activity and the other offering more psychotherapy. The activity-orientated programme was found to be significantly more effective with respect to a wide range of symptoms such as, decision making, use of leisure time, self-esteem and vocational adjustment.

Sports and games

The fashion for healthy physical activities, from jogging to aerobics, has also been reflected in occupational therapy departments. A range of activities can be encompassed here – on the sports side we might be involved in swimming (perhaps at the local baths), gym exercises, badminton and even team sports such as volley ball. On the games side we offer drama-type games (e.g. charades), quizzes (e.g. general knowledge), board games (e.g. *Trivial Pursuits*) and group activities such as bingo. Again the way the activities are structured greatly varies the end results. Bingo, for example, can be used as a way of teaching number/letter recognition, to encourage interaction (e.g. if participants share a card) or simply for fun. Whether competitive or not, sports or games offer enjoyment, opportunities for challenge, group interaction and they can be developed for leisure.

The positive impact of physical exercise on psychological well-being has been well researched. Moore and Bracegirdle (1994), for example, compared the psychological well-being and happiness of 15 elderly women who had undergone a 6-week exercise programme with that of a control group of 20 women. The women who had exercised, experienced a significant improvement in their feelings of happiness demonstrating an association between physical exercise and mental health. For other research references on this subject I recommend the literature review offered by Bracegirdle (1996).

Reminiscence therapy

In contrast to reality orientation, reminiscence therapy offers older people the opportunity to share memories and discuss how times have changed, and as such, it can be regarded more as a social activity. A range of slides, pictures and equipment are available for use, with the precaution of ensuring the patients are brought back to the present day at the end of the session. A useful textbook for reference covering this area is Coleman (1986).

THEORY INTO PRACTICE

Example activity evaluation: *Dance*

Value
1. Enjoyable/fun.
2. Socialising value of mixing with others (and possibly touching).
3. Promotes awareness of body movement and posture.
4. Stimulating, activating.
5. Can promote health, circulation, physical well-being, etc.
6. Sensory integration programmes.
7. Easily graded to suit any age group and skill level.

Ways of adapting
1. Activity itself – aerobics, old-time dance, jazz dance, disco dance, movement to music, Medau, mirroring, etc.
2. Complexity of steps.
3. Individual, partnership or group dancing.
4. New learning versus old skills.

Considerations
1. Resources – often need a skilled/experienced teacher.
2. Health risk, e.g. overexertion in aerobics or contraindications for heart/lung problems.
3. Special clothes/shoes required.
4. People may be overly conscious of their body shape, or have problems in touching others/being touched.

Activities involving communication and sharing

Communication and sharing with others can be incorporated into almost any activity, though most often they fall under the guise of 'groupwork'. Group members are encouraged to share their experiences and provide each other with mutual support and encouragement. Often the format of the activity is determined by the theoretical framework used, as seen when comparing dramatherapy (based on psychodynamic ideas) and social skills training (based on cognitive-behavioural principles). For a more in-depth exploration of the application of groupwork in occupational therapy, see Finlay (1993, 1996).

Discussion groups
These are handled in many ways, where aims, structure/format and the therapist role can all be adapted. For example, if we consider structured discussion, at one level, we can have a straightforward 'hat discussion' (hat passed round containing topic suggestions on slips of paper). At another level, more personal sharing can

be promoted by reading out and discussing the problem page/Agony Aunt letters in magazines.

The research by McDermott (1988) mentioned above demonstrated that the discussion based activity groups and verbal groups were beneficial for learning in that they promoted more discussion of feelings than craft-type groups.

Dramatherapy

This term encompasses remedial drama, socio-drama, role-play, psychodrama, and contains a wide range of activities, including games, action scenarios and group communication exercises. From its essentially humanistic base it can offer much to any age group and ability level, providing it is well handled. Some exercises may seem 'threatening' or 'childish' with inhibitions and resistances from group members, preventing movement. If taken slowly, however, and at a suitable level, the dramatherapy slot in the programme, with its emphasis on 'play', 'acting out' and group processes, can be the central pivot of therapy. One recommended text in this area is Jennings (1987).

Social skills training

This technique is sometimes confused with life skills education used with people with learning disabilities and with dramatherapy. In its purest use, however, social skills training is a cognitive behavioural technique designed to teach, systematically, elements of social behaviour (verbal, non-verbal, assertion, etc.). People who benefit may never have acquired the skills (e.g. people with learning disabilities), or had the skills once and lost them (e.g. institutionalised patients), or have the skills but lack the confidence to apply them (e.g. anxious individuals).

The practical emphasis on 'doing' and step-by-step learning of skills via role play, modelling, feedback, etc., make social skills training a particularly relevant technique to use in occupational therapy. Special sensitivity is needed, however, to tread the line between imposing one's own standards of behaviour and facilitating the development of new or different behaviours in someone who wants to change. Two useful texts in this area are Ellis and Whittington (1981), which lays out the theory; and Hutchings, Comins and Offiler (1991), which offers practical activity suggestions.

Anxiety management groups

Anxiety management groups are often presented as a 'course' and involves a closed group over a set number of weeks (commonly 10–12 sessions). The course consists of a number of treatment activities including education, groupwork, role play, relaxation exercises, etc. See Table 6.1 for a summary of the different areas of focus and type of treatment intervention. A more in-depth account of anxiety management is offered in Keable (1996).

Table 6.1 Anxiety management

Focus (anxiety component)	Treatment intervention
Cognition (e.g. negative thoughts)	(1) *Educating* the person about the nature of anxiety (about how different components can be natural/positive and how to 'spot and stop' the anxiety spiral). (2) *Cognitive restructuring* to encourage the person to stop negative thoughts/talk/anticipatory anxiety and to think more positively.
Behaviour (e.g. avoidance of anxiety provoking stimuli)	(3) *Systematic desensitisation* (or other structured and graded approaches) to unlearn avoidance behaviour. (4) *Role play* to practise specific skills and coping strategies for particular situations (such as an interview).
Physiology (e.g. autonomic responses)	(5) *Relaxation* [e.g. Jacobson's Progressive Muscular method or Mitchell's (1977) specific muscle group focus] and applied relaxation (e.g. what to do when sitting in a public place). (6) *Relaxing activities* (like going swimming, listening to music, doing yoga, playing squash, etc.). The individual is encouraged to find what works best for them and do it on a regular basis.

THEORY INTO PRACTICE

Example activity evaluation: *'Trust Games'*

Value
1. Group cohesion and working together.
2. Relaxing and pleasant sensations.
3. Trusting others physically promotes emotional trust.
4. Physical risk-taking promotes emotional risk-taking
5. Enjoyable/fun.

Ways of adapting
1. Activity itself – group lifts, swaying in a circle, fallbacks, run 'n' jump, blind walks, robots, etc.
2. Amount of risk and/or support.
3. Partnerships and different groupings.

Considerations
1. Physical safety, e.g. strained backs are common with poor lifting techniques. Careful instructions are necessary, plus accurate calculations of numbers of people needed.
2. Emotional safety, e.g. patient may be dropped or not handled sensitively. Whilst this may not be physically damaging, a sense of trust will not be developed. The

therapist needs to feel that the group members will handle each other gently. The therapist may need to be more directive, stepping in to take control in order to pre-empt any insensitive handling.
3. Contracts can be useful, e.g. (a) being 'responsible for your own body' or (b) not forcing anyone.
4. Correct clothing important.
5. Some members may be overly conscious of their weight or body or have inhibitions about touch.

Psychotherapy activities

These highly specialised activities arise mainly from the psychodynamic school, and focus on facilitating the expression and exploration of feelings. The activities can be more analytically based, emphasising unconscious conflict and symbols, or more humanistically orientated where self-awareness and growth are the end goals.

Psychodrama

This dramatic technique, pioneered by Moreno (1953), can be a powerful tool. Individuals enact/re-enact life scenes in an effort to explore their emotions, unconscious needs and relationships, both real and fantasy. The components of any psychodrama are: the stage (where life scenes are re-enacted), protagonist (person at centre of drama), director (therapist), auxiliary egos (group members who act the protagonists' family members, etc.), and the audience who respond and evaluate. Specific techniques are utilised, such as role play and role reversal, using the 'empty chair', and 'soliloquy'. Like all psychotherapy, skill, experience and some training is necessary before taking on a leader/director role.

Non-directive play therapy

The use of play in therapy can be separated into non-directive play therapy versus directive play therapy. These can be further sub-divided according to their different theoretical commitments, for instance psychoanalytical or developmental approaches. For a fuller analysis of these different variants, see Jeffrey (1995).

Non-directive playtherapy is a technique, pioneered by Virginia Axline (1971), which has been used as a model for many occupational therapists working in child psychiatry. Briefly, a child is offered the free use of a playroom, to play out feelings, needs and fantasies. Playing out the feelings enables the child to begin to understand and so control them. The therapist attempts to be non-judgmental, and lets the child lead, acting mainly as a mirror to reflect back the play's content to the child. Accepting the child, whatever feelings are displayed, enables the child to accept him or herself.

Projective activities

Art, drama, pottery, poetry, music are all creative activities which have been used

in a psychotherapeutic way to help individuals to gain insight into their inner conflicts and explore their feelings. The key process underlying any projective
activity involves individuals in 'projecting' or externalising their inner feelings
outwards, onto a creative object (e.g. paper). As Waller expresses it, 'image making in the presence of the therapist may enable a client to get in touch with early
repressed feelings ... and that the ensuing art object may act as a container for
powerful emotions that cannot be easily expressed' (Waller, 1993, p. 3). When
these projective activities take place in a group setting additional benefits can be
gained, for instance mutual support. For a fuller account of occupational therapy
and group psychotherapy, see Blair (1990).

THEORY INTO PRACTICE

Example activity evaluation: *Projective Art*

Value
1. Self-awareness, insight.
2. Expression and exploration of emotions or catharsis.
3. Group communication, sharing, cohesion, support.
4. Enjoyable.

Note there are two different stages involved with doing projective art: doing the art
work and then talking about it afterwards. The art process itself (e.g. painting a picture on 'how I feel') can offer some cathartic release. Talking about it afterwards
(discussion or psychotherapy format) can help individuals to further their feelings
and enables group members to give each other support. Different therapists place a
different emphasis on the two stages – some prefer the doing, others the talk.

Ways of adapting
1. Extend the time for either 'doing' or 'talking'
2. Activity itself – free self-expression, fun games, painting to music, painting to a
   theme, interpretative analysis, etc.
3. Vary themes and titles, e.g. 'How I see myself now ... in 5 years', 'my family',
   'schizophrenia', 'happiness', What I like/dislike', 'what alcohol means to me ...'
4. Media used – clay, paint, finger-paint, collage, rollerbrushes, etc.

Considerations
1. Emotional safety/trust within the group essential.
2. Emphasise the importance of free spontaneous art as opposed to being concerned
   about the artistic end-product.
3. Contraindications: (a) dangers of stirrings up feelings as the activity can be emotionally powerful; (b) over-interpretation can be offensive or simply wrong; (c)
   may reinforce fantasy, confusion, with, for example, those with thought disorder.
4. Decide between running a more analytical/psychodynamic art group where interpretation (e.g. symbols) is desirable versus a more humanistic approach where
   self-awareness and growth are the end goals.

Activity analysis

One of the key skills utilised by occupational therapists is the ability to analyse the component parts of an activity. This enables us to select meaningful activity and use it purposefully to enhance a person's growth and functioning. The step-by-step analysis can be laborious, but it is important to do, until the therapist feels familiar with both the nature of the activity and its potential as a treatment medium.

What do we analyse?

Activity analysis usually occurs in two stages. First, we try to understand the *intrinsic* aspects of the activity itself. Then we analyse how the activity can be utilised (i.e. graded and adapted) towards a *therapeutic* end (what Hagedorn, 1996 refers to as 'applied analysis').

Young and Quinn (1992) suggest that activities can be analysed in terms of (a) the permanent, unchanging requirements intrinsic to the activity (e.g. sensori-motor and cognitive demands), (b) permanent, changing requirements (such as space, equipment, materials and cost), and (c) social and cultural perceptions of the performances of an activity (e.g. expectations related to gender, age and ethnicity).

Occupational therapists probe activity at all levels investigating:

- The steps, procedures and processes involved.
- Materials and tools required.
- Motions and sequences involved.
- The environmental context.
- The results of the process.
- Its cultural and social meanings.

We look at all these aspects, paying particular attention to how demanding the activity is in terms of a person's functioning in the following areas:

- *Physical* – what type of movements are required: fine, gross, repetitive, aggressive? What kind of tolerance and strength is needed?
- *Sensory/perceptual* – what visual, tactile, proprioceptive aspects are involved?
- *Cognitive* – how much concentration, memory, intellectual ability, abstract thought, etc., is needed?
- *Emotional* – does the activity ease expression of feelings? Does it satisfy needs? Is it stimulating? Is it intrinsically/extrinsically motivating?
- *Social* – what level of communication skill is required? How much sharing and co-operative behaviour is expected?

In addition to analysing the demands of the activity on the individual, we build up a picture of the inherent nature of the activity. Demands, may be noted, such as: 'this activity needs attention to detail', or 'some amount of tolerance to dirt is required', or 'there are cultural assumptions behind this activity making it unsuitable for certain groups'. We then marry this information with the individual's needs, ability and motivation.

Why analyse an activity?

Having broken down an activity into its steps and demands, we can utilise the activity's potential to restore or maintain function. This can be seen clearly in four ways.

Firstly, we analyse an activity *to determine if a patient/client can do it*. For example, the apparently simple task of making a collage may not be so easily achieved if it takes place in a group setting, and the individual concerned operates below a parallel group level in terms of Mosey's group interaction skill levels. Another example is that we might feel more confident about encouraging a person to use a pottery wheel if we assess he or she has: some standing tolerance; co-ordination; familiarity with claywork; and some perseverance while learning a new skill. (Note that an increase in skill level can only be achieved if some aspect of the activity is slightly beyond the person's ability, thus creating a goal to strive towards.)

Secondly, we also break down activity into smaller steps and sub-tasks for *teaching purposes*. An accurate preliminary analysis allows us to consider if there is a logical progression or if any steps need to be simplified or eliminated. The process of teaching someone how to make a coil pot, for example, might involve a step-by-step progression of:

1. Therapist demonstrates showing basic idea and result.
2. Patient/client makes base after another demonstration and with physical and verbal promoting.
3. Patient/client practises making coils with advice.
4. Patient/client makes coils and applies to pot using slip, after instruction and demonstration.
5. Therapist demonstrates how to finish off coil pot.
6. Patient/client makes another pot with minimal instruction given.

Each stage of the process contains its own skill levels and needs to be carried out in sequence if the end-product is to be successful. Throughout the teaching it is also important to consider the patient's cognitive ability as well as his or her needs for reward or encouragement.

Thirdly, we also analyse activities in order to identify what aspects need to be *adapted* or altered in order to ensure a useful experience suited to the person's functional ability. Thus a person who finds working in a group difficult, and is unable to join in a group collage, may be asked to make an individual collage which is later added to the larger one. Alternatively, the individual learning to cook, but who is unable to read, may need picture recipe cards instead of written ones.

Finally, we analyse activity in order to *grade it* to bring about change. For example, we can identify which components need to be made more demanding, thereby stretching function. An example of this can be seen in woodwork where treatment might move from simple sanding to making intricate sculpture puzzles, thus encouraging the patient/client towards higher amounts of concentration or attention to detail.

6.3 ACTIVITY IN TREATMENT

One mistake occupational therapists can make when using activities arises when we feel confident about the value of an activity and thus assume its therapeutic effect. An example of this is the patient who has the problem of poor eye contact and is encouraged to play a game of 'wink-murder' because it utilises eye contact. Another patient, with poor concentration, is given dressmaking, as it requires some mental application. On careful examination, though, it is clear these activities will only prove beneficial as part of a graded programme. Thus, wink murder is only useful (for eye contact) if the person concerned finds it slightly difficult to do, and this requires the occupational therapist to carefully adjust the demands of the game. Likewise, people with poor concentration who engage in dressmaking will need regular encouragement by the occupational therapist, enabling them to attend to the task. It is not the dressmaking itself which improves concentration, but *how it is applied*.

Consider the five case illustrations below of how activities may be applied as part of the treatment and problem-solving process. The examples also show how both the therapist's approach and the process of structuring of the environment are fundamentally linked to the grading of an activity.

6.4 CASE ILLUSTRATIONS

Case illustration 6.1: Michael

Problem	Poor task performance skills
Activity	Woodwork
Grading	Increasing the demands and complexity of task

Michael, aged 40, has had repeated admissions to hospital with a diagnosis of schizophrenia. His basic task performance was poor, probably resulting from a combination of cognitive deficit stemming from his illness, passive behaviour due to institutionalisation, and the sedating effects of his medication. A concrete task for which Michael expressed an interest was woodwork.

Stage 1: Basic task and quick results
With his concentration being so poor initially, the occupational therapist encouraged Michael to make something which could be completed fairly quickly and

which required a minimal amount of skill. Over the first week several tasks were completed, such as varnishing a ready-made stool and sanding/polishing a bread-board for the ward. These activities required the minimum of instruction, and were repetitive enough to allow Michael's attention to wander whilst still producing constructive end-products which he could feel pleasure about.

Stage 2: Increased task demands

As Michael settled into the routines of the new area, more complex tasks were introduced involving more complex instructions and which took longer amounts of time. First, he made a plant trough out of pre-cut strips of wood which he then painted. Later, with the occupational therapist's help, he made an intricate chess-board requiring careful cutting and staining of the wood.

Stage 3: Discharge

Michael pursued his new interest in woodwork when he was discharged to attend a day centre three times a week.

Case illustration 6.2: June

Problem	Lack of self-confidence
Activity	Jewellery making with metalwork
Grading	Early success experience leading on to increased task demands and difficulties as therapist gradually reduces supportive assistance

Discussion point. Lack of confidence is a problem that most of us have in some area or other and it is usually situation(s) specific. Activity, and 'doing' treatments, can only problem solve successfully if the confidence problem involves the individual's ability to do or to achieve, in that particular area. In other words, a house-wife may gain confidence from learning to cook and sew, *if* she feels inadequate in her role. However, if she has a negative view of herself as a result of being abused, such activities are not likely to make a significant impact. Having said that, a tangible success experience can result in positive self-feelings and may be the start of some longer term work. [A word of caution though: If the experience is too easy, negative feelings can be confirmed and the activity can prove destructive. So care must be taken to grade both the activity and the therapist's role sensitively.]

June, a 23-year-old unemployed woman, greatly lacked confidence in her abilities. She had started several college courses, but either failed or gave up. She felt 'use-less', but agreed to give occupational therapy a chance.

Stage 1: Introducing the activity

June expressed an interest in jewellery making, though also said 'I won't be able to make anything as nice as those samples'. The occupational therapist suggested she give it a week, and that she first learn the basic skills. This approach was adopted to avoid being overly praising (as June was likely to negate compliments or reassurances) and also to encourage June to be more realistic about her skills.

Stage 2: Teach basic skills and provide success experience

The occupational therapist taught June a simple and quick method of beading and bending a piece of wire to make an earring. June was provided with a range of examples and ideas, and was encouraged to 'have a go'. The results were successful, came quickly and provided an immediate reward. June could not deny she could produce some basic, pretty jewellery.

Stage 3: Increase demands of activity

June's initial good feelings about her achievement soon diminished and she began to put down her skill, saying the task was too easy. The occupational therapist agreed, and showed her a much more complicated method requiring new welding and enamelling techniques. The occupational therapist was actively involved, both encouraging June and supervising her closely in order to pre-empt any failure.

Stage 4: Reduce therapist support

As June's ability and confidence grew, the occupational therapist withdrew both her help and encouragement. The occupational therapist began to 'allow' June to use her own ideas, and make mistakes, and also more realistically gave constructive criticisms. Thus June could feel unqualified confidence from her results.

Case illustration 6.3: Kathy

Problem	Anxiety
Activity	Anxiety management group
Grading	Occurs through the course of 12 supportive/educational sessions where the therapist increasingly encourages group members to support each other and implement their own problem solving as their knowledge and skill increases

Kathy is a 32-year-old secretary. She had begun to feel extremely anxious at work, though she did not know why. She was finding it hard to concentrate at work and so was making mistakes which worried her further as she normally had high standards. She felt she was failing at everything and she lacked confidence in her judgements. Kathy became particularly frightened after experiencing a full blown 'panic attack'. On assessment, the therapist discovered that Kathy lived with her husband (unemployed) and there was a suggestion that she was being physically abused by him. Despite this, Kathy expressed wanting children 'before it is too late'.

Stage 1: Education about anxiety and relaxation techniques

Kathy joined the newly formed anxiety management group. The emphasis in the first couple of sessions was learning how to contain and cope with her anxiety. She learned how her negative thoughts and anxiety about anxiety, provoked an anxiety spiral. She practised different relaxation techniques in order to identify which worked best for her.

Stage 2: Support and sharing in the group

Kathy had begun to feel her anxiety was under control and that she could cope with it. Through the support and sharing in the group she realised that her anxiety was largely linked to marital stress.

Stage 3: Discharge planning
Kathy gained confidence in managing her own anxiety by teaching and supporting others. Her final 'homework' task was to begin marital counselling sessions with 'Relate'. Once these sessions had begun she was discharged from the group and given a follow-up appointment for 3 months later.

Case illustration 6.4: Clyde

Problem	Identity and work conflicts
Activity	Counselling and groupwork
Grading	Not particularly relevant – group process evolved over time

Clyde is a 35-year-old accountant. He was under a great deal of stress at work and went to his GP for insomnia and palpitations. The GP referred him on to the occupational therapist in the Community Mental Health team for stress management. On assessment the therapist discovered Clyde's work was the problem area where he was irritable and experiencing interpersonal difficulties. He felt angry/upset as he had expected a good promotion but had been 'passed over again'. He felt his bosses in the firm were racist (Clyde has a white Scottish mother and a black African father).

Stage 1: One-to-one supportive counselling
The therapist's main intervention was to see Clyde once a week for one-to-one supportive counselling. The main focus was on exploring how Clyde could cope better with his work tensions.

Stage 2: Joining a men's group
After 4 weeks of exploratory one-to-one sessions, Clyde was encouraged to join a supportive Men's Group which the occupational therapist ran. The group consisted of seven men (including the therapist) who were between the ages of 22 and 37. They used the opportunity to explore issues concerning: work, relationships, gender, sexuality, power and racism. During one session, the group specifically helped Clyde by practising a role-play of how Clyde could tackle the racism/promotion issue with his boss.

Case illustration 6.5: Darren

Problem	Hyper-activity and poor concentration
Activity	Cooking
Grading	Increase social distractions and demands of the task

Darren, aged 12, had a history of being overactive which impaired both his concentration and social skills. His behaviour tended to get out of control which had resulted in him being excluded from school on several occasions. Twice weekly remedial therapy sessions were implemented utilising both structured learning activities and cooking.

Stage 1: Quick cookery tasks

Initially the therapist worked one-to-one with Darren doing quick cookery tasks. For instance Darren would make a small cake using a cake mix. He responded positively to these times and gained particular pleasure consuming the products at the end of the session!

Stage 2: Longer cookery tasks

Once Darren could contain himself and concentrate on tasks lasting between 15 and 30 minutes, he began to cook more complicated things. At his request he cooked a cake from 'scratch', and produced an entire lunch of fish fingers and baked beans.

Stage 3: Group work

Darren agreed to let two other boys join him. Initially he found having others in the group difficult (he was inclined to be aggressive and his attention span was poor). As he began to feel more comfortable, he was given the responsibility of 'being in charge' and he rose to the occasion. The group celebrated their last session by cooking a special lunch for all the children in the unit (no mean feat!).

CONCLUSION

This chapter has explored the social basis of occupations and how we use activities in treatment. Occupational therapists use a variety of activities in therapy, and in order to apply them effectively we need to appreciate their specific properties and limitations. The therapeutic potential of an activity emerges when it is carefully structured and graded for the individuals concerned. Thus our belief in the healing power of activities comes both from its intrinsic value and from the skill with which it is applied. Using illustrative case studies, the next chapter continues to explore how occupational therapists focus on occupation and use activities therapeutically.

Discussion questions

1. Illustrate how culture influences occupations and our use of therapy activities.
2. The therapeutic value of occupational therapy activities arises from the grading process rather than any inherent value of the activity itself. Explain this statement.
3. What aspects of an activity need to be analysed and why?
4. How can woodwork (or another activity) be graded to improve (a) task performance skills and (b) social interaction skills?
5. Is work rehabilitation largely irrelevant in today's economic climate?
6. Does the use of counselling in occupational therapy go against our role as it does not have an activity base?

Implementation of treatment   7

Any discussion on the implementation of treatment must seek to synthesise all aspects of the occupational therapy process from assessment to evaluation, as discussed in previous chapters. I have attempted to achieve this synthesis via 12 contrasting case studies chosen to illustrate the diversity of our occupational therapy practice. Each case illustration is intended to indicate both the different types of patients/clients we treat and the different approaches to treatment we adopt. Though these case illustrations are not verbatim accounts of actual patients'/clients' records, the material for them is drawn largely from my clinical experience, and so reflects the kinds of problems and treatments encountered in occupational therapy.

In these examples I have tried to demonstrate: our wide eclectic base; short- and long-term aspects of treatment; hospital and community care; our clinical reasoning; and some of the issues/complexities that can arise as part of the therapy process. I have not tried to offer a representative sample of our work as it varies so much. I have also not explored the many frustrations, disappointments and anxieties we experience, though the discussion sections touch on some of these issues. The case examples offered are necessarily selective guides to the scope and depth of our work but I hope they will generate ideas for practice and discussion. For instance, if you disagree with the treatment described, what would you offer? Why?

To assist ease of reading and comparisons to be made, I have organised all the case illustrations under the standard headings of: summary of history; team strategy; initial occupational therapy assessment; treatment planning; progress of treatment; and discussion. I have not produced discussion questions at the end of the chapter. In place of these, reflect on the following questions as you go through each case illustration:

1. What is the key occupational therapy role identifiable in each study?
2. Select an alternative theoretical framework. How would this change the treatment applied?

3. In your view, how should the problems identified in each study be prioritised and handled?
4. How could the occupational therapist grade each suggested activity to effectively meet the associated aims/objectives?
5. Would any of the individuals be treated differently in your clinical set-up? How and Why?
6. None of the case illustrations mention the individual's race or ethnicity. Would it change your treatment if you knew a person was, for instance of AfroCarribean or Asian descent? Would treatment change if the person's religion was indicated?

Case illustration 7.1: Catherine

Key issues   Retirement and alcohol abuse

Summary of history

Catherine, a 68-year-old woman, lives alone in an attractive house with her two cats. She retired 8 years ago from her job as a librarian at the local university (a job she had held for 20 years). Since that time she has become isolated and inactive. She has few friends and no family near by. Catherine has a long-standing history of being a heavy drinker but she kept it largely under control whilst she was working. She now tends to drink alcohol throughout the day – as she says, 'It helps me feel good'. Catherine's alcohol abuse came to light after a fall where she fractured her femur. Having admitted her problem to herself, she went to her GP for help in tackling it, who then referred her to the Community Mental Health Unit (Substance Abuse team).

Team strategy

The team agreed that the likely focus of treatment should be on helping Catherine to develop some alternative, meaningful occupations and so she was allocated to the occupational therapist. The psychiatrist was to assist with medication if requested/required.

Initial occupational therapy assessment

Two preliminary interviews (home visits) were undertaken. The occupational therapist first explored Catherine's view of the alcohol problem and her motivation to manage it. The OPHI was used to structure the interview where Catherine compared her life from 8 years ago to now. Several self-rating assessments were employed alongside to explore her roles, pattern of daily activities, interests and values.

Assessment revealed that whilst Catherine wanted to manage her drinking, she did not want to give it up entirely. She realised, however, she would need some extra support for controlling her intake. She agreed with the therapist that her main need was to find and develop some meaningful occupations – ones that could productively fill the void that had opened up with her retirement. She expressed interest in swimming on a regular basis (to get back into shape physically) and returning to creative writing (a hobby she had always loved and enjoyed prior to retirement).

Treatment planning

Aims/objectives	Treatment methods
1. Implement a controlled drinking regime with support.	(a) Use of contract and review of daily drinking habits (recording intake and associated feelings/events in a diary).
	(b) Group work – weekly supportive psychotherapy group for 'ex' and 'controlled' drinkers.
2. Set goals towards implementing a new activity programme.	Range of activities engaged in:
	(a) Swimming at least three times a week.
	(b) Creative writing at least once a week.
	(c) Join a new club/class.

Progress of treatment

Catherine was highly motivated and responded well to her new activity programme and having the active professional input. She found the diary writing difficult to maintain but insight-giving. Initially she had been shocked to realise how much she did drink which provided her an extra spur to treatment. Through her diary she learned about her stress points and 'drinking triggers', and so she was enabled to take more control of her behaviour.

She found the groupwork threatening/stressful and after the first session was reluctant to return. The occupational therapist negotiated with her to give it a try for 1 month (four sessions). Catherine complied. She soon found the group to be both supportive and instructive, and she eventually became a long-standing attender.

In terms of her activities, Catherine joined an over-50s swim club which she enjoyed for both the activity and the social element. She also signed up for a creative writing evening class which became the highlight of her week. On her discharge interview Catherine said she was working on producing a volume of short stories and poetry.

Overall, the treatment had proved extremely successful in terms of facilitating new meaningful occupations. The treatment was not without its problem times however. For one thing, Catherine lapsed and broke her controlled drinking regime on two separate occasions (which resulted in withdrawing from her 'new life' for several weeks). The important lesson for her to learn was that she could get back on track when she had similar lapses in the future.

Discussion

Catherine's treatment raises several issues related to clients' motivation that frequently crop up in the context of client-centred practice. First, for Catherine's treatment to have any chance of success, she needed to be motivated to carry out the controlled drinking programme. Had she not wanted to change (at some level) and had not been prepared to engage actively in goal setting, any attempt at treatment would have been fairly pointless. The real battle for our patients/clients is often the first one – of them acknowledging they have a problem with which they want to grapple.

A second issue relates to the notion that client-centred practice respects clients' own choice and autonomy. In this case the occupational therapist negotiated with Catherine to attend a group which she was reluctant to do. It could be argued that the therapist's approach was inconsistent with client-centred philosophy. The key to this dilemma is to focus on the therapist–client *partnership*. There is a difference between coercion and negotiation (where the therapist explains the potential gains of the group and acknowledges the client's understandable anxieties). Importantly, the final decision of whether or not to attend had to reside with Catherine.

Case illustration 7.2: Sally

Key issues   Anxiety management and return to work

Summary of history
Sally, 32 years old, was admitted to an acute admission unit with a diagnosis of anxiety neurosis. She said she could not cope any more with her panic attacks and tension headaches. She even blacked out once, apparently from stress, during her work as a stylist in a hairdressing salon. Sally lives with her boyfriend and their 7-year-old daughter. She appears to be experiencing tensions in her relationship with her boyfriend.

Team strategy
On the ward she was given both medication and opportunities to express her feelings. The social worker became involved in doing some 'marital' counselling. A nurse and the occupational therapist worked jointly to organise an anxiety-management programme.

Initial occupational therapy assessment
On interview she presented as being well-dressed and groomed, though anxious about her looks, as she kept apologising for her tearful blotchy face and the fact that she had not put on any makeup. She stressed that she was particularly concerned that her panic attacks had been interfering with her work. Over the previous few months she had grown increasingly anxious that she was making mistakes and is being criticised for them. As a result, Sally was checking clients' hair excessively and this had resulted in their loss of confidence in her.

Treatment planning

Aims/objectives	Treatment methods
1. To learn anxiety-management strategies and gain confidence to cope with her anxiety.	Anxiety-management course covering: (a) Educational aspects of the nature of anxiety and cognitive restructuring (e.g. 'I can cope'). (b) Relaxation and yoga classes. (c) Group discussions on anxiety (d) Some music activities used for relaxation.

| 2. In the long term, to return to work gradually (where she will be able to apply her new coping strategies). | Initially build her confidence by encouraging her to do hair on the ward in a beauty care group. Later implement a graded return to work with some limited follow-up. |

Progress of treatment

Sally was treated as an in-patient for 1 week and as an out-patient for a further month. In the latter period she made a successful reintegration into her work, aided by supportive colleagues. The social worker continued to see Sally and her partner, as more fundamental problems seemed situated there. From the occupational therapy point of view, Sally gained from the practical anxiety-management input and the support she gained from other group members.

Discussion

In this study, the occupational therapist adopted an occupational performance model where Sally's work role functioning was the central concern. To treat her, the therapist employed cognitive-behavioural techniques (seen in the anxiety management programme and the graded return to work).

It is possible to frame Sally's treatment in contrasting ways. For instance, if we adopted a more humanistic focus, we might view the beauty care activities as a way of raising her self-esteem (through success experience and being valued by others) and learning the relaxation techniques as a way of giving her a greater sense of control.

Case illustration 7.3: George

Key issues   Chronic schizophrenia and rehabilitation

Summary of history

George, a 42-year-old man, attended a day hospital for long-term rehabilitation and support. He had his first schizophrenic breakdown when he was in his 20s and since then had spent a significant proportion of his life in the local hospital. Whilst maintained on long-term medication, his behaviour and skills show evidence of institutionalisation. His referral to the day hospital was an attempt to maintain his skills and life in the community, prevent in-patient admission, and provide him with some productive role during the day. He lives with his sister (and her family) who also require some support and a break from George in the day.

Team strategy

The doctor monitored the medication and involved the family in some family therapy. The community psychiatric nurse undertook regular home visits to monitor George, provide medication, and give the family support. The psychologist was involved in setting up a range of behavioural programmes including social skills training and token economy. The occupational therapist's was concerned with George's occupational performance and skills (self-care, task performance and social).

Initial occupational therapy assessment

The priority problems identified, from observing George in activities and carrying out the standardised FPR assessment included:

1. Task performance – George's skills were poor, i.e. poor concentration (less than 10 minutes on routine work task), limited problem-solving ability, difficulty in following verbal instructions and lack of attention to detail.
2. General behaviour – compliance, dependence and passivity in evidence. Social skills reduced, especially difficulties with posture, eye contact and initiating conversation
3. On the strengths side – George was friendly when approached and his self-care presentation was relatively good. This was likely to be due in part to his sister's influence. He was also motivated to attend the day hospital and responded positively to both praise and concrete rewards such as tokens.

Treatment planning

Aims/objectives	Treatment methods
1. To practice productive work role behaviour towards increasing his sense of competence, esteem/status and improving task performance skills.	Light industrial work, grading, amount of concentration required, responsibility, etc. Consider for the long term the possibility of day centre attendance.
2. To develop a greater sense of self, initiative, autonomy and responsibility.	(a) Day hospital environment and consistent team approach. (b) Success experience in work. (c) Use of own behavioural target setting (e.g. 'by the end of the week I will have achieved …').
3. To develop social skills and widen leisure opportunities.	(a) Once-weekly social skills group. (b) Twice-weekly general social activities group within day hospital. (c) Encouragement to take up evening activities and holidays, both with family and outside.
4. To develop productive domestic role.	Twice-weekly lunch cooking group.

Progress of treatment

George regularly attended the day hospital over a period of 2 years, during which time he gradually moved on to a local day centre (with the community psychiatric nurse maintaining contact). In the first year, treatment was geared to improving specific task skills in the industrial therapy workshop. The fortnightly self and supervisor appraisal and goal-setting interview (behavioural emphasis) was a significant part of his progress. He was promoted in his work position, which did much for his self-esteem.

The latter part of George's rehabilitation focused on his involvement and role at home (trying to increase his level of responsibility taken). To this end he learned how to cook two set meals which his family enjoyed. George increasingly took responsibility for these two meals for the family once or twice a week – a development much appreciated by his sister. George made some significant gains during his stay at the hospital, but remained vulnerable, needing a sheltered, structured environment.

Discussion

Any discussion of George's rehabilitation must include a recognition of the team approach found characteristically in many day hospitals. In these instances it is often difficult to identify a special occupational therapy role – indeed, we may sometimes feel confused when we see nurses managing industrial therapy units, or the psychologists running the social skills group! This poses the question of whether or not this is beneficial to the patients. Most team enthusiasts would say we should not defensively guard our role, but work together, drawing on our own particular skills (be they personal or professional skills).

Whilst role-blurring is an increasingly common phenomenon, the occupational therapist's specific role can still be understood in terms of the focus on a person's occupational (work, social or domestic) performance. In some units the occupational therapist may emphasise work roles and use industrial/clerical work or heavy workshop type activities. If the occupational therapists favour a more domestic line, they may use a half-way house or employ home management activities. Many of the more socially orientated therapists will explore the use of leisure and community facilities. All of these are a legitimate use of our time and skills – and given how important we think these aspects are, is it surprising that other professionals agree?

Case illustration 7.4: Steve

Key issues   Head injury, assessing and treating cognitive function

Summary of history

Steve, 19 years old, sustained a head injury following a motor cycle accident. Initially he required intensive care as he was confused, disorientated and unable to carry out any self-care. After 3 weeks his functioning was greatly improved, though he was left with some residual damage. He had some physical problems (i.e. weakness, tremor and co-ordination difficulty down his right side) plus some motor dyspraxia and cognitive deficits. He was transferred to a rehabilitation ward for intensive therapy (first as an in-patient, then latterly as a day-patient).

Steve was in his first year of university doing a building degree. He was both popular and an academically strong student. He shared a house with some friends and had an active social life. His accident required him to put university life on hold and he returned to live with his parents for his recuperation.

Team strategy

The physiotherapist worked on Steve's mobility/co-ordination problems whilst the occupational therapist focused on assessing and improving his dyspraxia and cognitive difficulties. The team envisaged Steve would need several months of treatment and rehabilitation, but they could not predict to what extent he would be able to return to his previous functioning.

Occupational therapy assessment

The occupational therapist carried out a range of assessments which resulted in the following findings:

Assessment	Findings
COTNAB to assess perceptual/ cognitive function.	Difficulties most apparent for: hidden figures, three-dimensional construction, block printing, dexterity, co-ordination, following written instructions. Slow performance for the above as well as sequencing and two-dimensional construction.
AMPS to assess skills related to ADL functioning – tasks used: toast and instant coffee; making a bed with a duvet.	Particular problems revealed (i.e. scores of 2) on: posture, mobility, co-ordination, strength and effort, energy, temporal organisation and adaptation. He was slow in performing the tasks and showed difficulties about accommodating/learning from experience.
Computer games (an activity he enjoyed) to observe general problem solving and concentration.	Concentration problems exposed (i.e. he could only attend to a game for about 10 minutes at a time whereas he used to play for hours); problem solving difficulties regarding abstract problems also apparent.
Occupational performance tasks (e.g. dressing, shaving) to assess personal ADL and safety.	Steve proved to be slow at these tasks but he managed them independently.

Treatment planning

Aims/objectives	Treatment methods
Early stage 1. Ensure independence in dressing/self-care. 2. Develop concentration and problem-solving. 3. Promote normal movement patterns for occupational performance tasks.	(a) Dressing practice and other ADL tasks. (b) Computer games (for increasing lengths of time starting with 15 minute slots and working up to 1 hour daily). (c) Twice weekly cooking group (including going to the shops and cooking a range of meals/snacks).

Middle stage

1. Develop 'normal' social interactions and movement patterns.
2. Continue to improve perceptual and cognitive functioning.

(a) Once weekly 'social gym' session (e.g. volley ball, team badminton, swimming at the local baths).
(b) Computer games and 'work' related to his university studies.

Late stage

1. Return (if possible) to building degree course having taken a year out.
2. Arrange to discuss with course tutor preparation for course and course work requirements.

(a) Computer work – revising and doing some old assignments/projects.
(b) Exercises in maths and technical drawing (house plans, etc.).

Progress of treatment

Steve worked doggedly at his rehabilitation as he was strongly motivated to return to his university course. He enjoyed all his computer games and used his computer time well to monitor improving function. On the therapist's advice he had monitored and recorded his performance daily (e.g. he measured his increasing game scores and the length of time he concentrated). Steve's gym sessions proved effective at both a physical and social level. The games helped with his balance/co-ordination, speeded up his reactions and encouraged him to 'lighten up' and have some fun with other group members. Steve did not enjoy the cooking sessions but he could see that they were useful for developing his functional ability.

Steve was discharged after 8 months of rehabilitation. The team (including Steve) felt he would be able to return to his university course, though he was to change to do an ordinary rather than honours degree. His physical functioning had improved significantly though he remained a touch slow both in movements and thinking. He retained some mild cognitive problems (e.g. his abstract thinking remained slightly impaired and he tended to be 'rule bound'). At a social level he appeared to have lost much of his old charm, sense of humour and ability to converse fluently. Steve recognised he had changed but was unable to identify what was different. Steve's mother was the one who seemed most disturbed by the personality changes and continuing impairment. In confidence, she confided to the occupational therapist, 'I have lost my son'.

Six months after discharge he returned for a follow-up review interview. The treatment team were pleased to hear Steve was coping with his course though he had to work long hours to keep up. Although he was experiencing some social isolation problems he felt pleased about his progress and hopeful for his future.

Discussion

Steve's case is a good illustration of the overlap between physical and psychosocial occupational therapy. Depending on the treatment context (e.g. type of rehabilitation unit), he could have been treated by an occupational therapist specialising in either neurology or liaison psychiatry (mental health practitioner who is brought into a general hospital setting as a 'consultant'). Occupational therapists are particularly well placed (given our dual training) to offer this kind of 'holistic' treatment where a person's long-term functioning related to physical, mental and social aspects are encompassed. Some occupational therapists would argue that we should be more involved in this kind of treatment and withdraw from short-term interventions in acute settings. What do you think?

Case illustration 7.5: Ed

Key issues   Acute manic episode of a chronic disorder and dilemmas of work rehabilitation

Summary of history

Ed, a 43-year-old man, was admitted to hospital with a diagnosis of 'schizo-affective disorder' and a history of manic episodes. On admission Ed was very 'high' with pressure of speech and a volatile temper. He had not slept or eaten for 5 days but was still 'buzzing around'. During this current manic episode he had spent £15 000 buying computers for his 'new' (not formed except in his head) business as a creative marketing expert. He was convinced he was a world-wide success. He was brought into hospital on a Section to be stabilised on medication. He did not mind this particularly as the hospital and staff were familiar to him, and he looked on them as friends with whom he could share his many ideas.

Ed's continuing mental illness has been destructive to his marriage (his wife left him 6 years ago) and has seriously impaired his work/social relationships. Ed has worked as a fifth form teacher at the local school for the past 15 years where he has a reputation for having been an excellent charismatic teacher. His recent reputation is more problematic however, as he has had two major breakdowns in 3 years. The school children and his colleagues have had to cope with some very odd behaviour and the fact that he has had extended periods off sick. Whilst his head of department has been supportive and understanding, his colleagues are reluctant to have him back.

Team strategy

The ward staff found him extremely difficult to contain as he reacted aggressively when any attempt was made to curb his behaviour. He was slightly calmer in the more 'normal' and quieter atmosphere of the Occupational Therapy Department. This was partly because he had 'fallen in love' with the Head Occupational Therapist and was content to sit and watch her work. She was also one of the few people (along with his Consultant and the Charge Nurse) from whom he would accept direction. He felt the senior staff were his 'equals'.

The team's short-term aim of treatment was to get Ed re-stabilised on medication and to try to contain his manic and aggressive behaviour. As far as possible, only the Charge Nurse, Consultant and Head Occupational Therapist had direct dealings with Ed to minimise the threat of violence. The occupational therapist (reluctantly) agreed to accept Ed in the Occupational Therapy Department each morning – partly to help quieten his behaviour and partly to monitor the effects of the medication.

Initial occupational therapy assessment

Ed was encouraged to engage in concrete activities in an effort to contain his behaviour. When interested in an activity, Ed was able to concentrate for up to 20 minutes. He needed prompting (and contracts involving the withdrawal of the privilege of coming to the department) to hold his enthusiasm in check. No other formal assessment was attempted at this stage as his behaviour was likely to change significantly once stabilised on medication.

Treatment planning

Aims/objectives	Treatment methods
Short term	
Engage in concrete task-orientated behaviour to develop concentration and reduce activity level.	Any activity which Ed could do by himself (quietly) with the occupational therapist monitoring him at a distance. Ed often chose an art activity. The OT encouraged him to do some printing.
Middle term	
Once stabilised on medication begin to return home (with support from the OT) and sort out business.	Home visits with support initially; later he would stay through the afternoon by himself.
Long term	
Prepare and carry out simulated lessons as part of a work hardening programme and work assessment to establish if it is realistic and appropriate to return	(a) Simulated teaching sessions. (b) High-level printing to assess concentration and task performance. (c) Discussion with the occupational therapist and doctor about managing the difficult return to work.

Progress of treatment

Initially, Ed's behaviour proved to be too disruptive and volatile for the Occupational Therapy Department and he was confined to the ward. After a couple of weeks he had calmed down sufficiently to join in some art and printing sessions and to develop concentration and ability to follow through concrete tasks.

After 7 weeks of admission, Ed's mental state became more stable and he was ready to begin to sort out problems at home. The occupational therapist (and another staff member) did a home visit with Ed. They found an appalling mess including computer equipment still new in boxes all over the place. Ed's task for the next few weeks was to clean and tidy his home; try to get refunds on the equipment; and sort out his correspondence, finances and many unpaid bills, etc. All of this was quite difficult for Ed to handle – not least because he was confronted by how 'mad' he had been and had not recognised it. He went home from the hospital each day. Sometimes the occupational therapist or another member of staff would go with him to give him some support. After a couple of weeks, the strain of this process began to tell. Ed became depressed and his home treatment had to be suspended temporarily. When he was ready he restarted his home programme and spent increasing periods of time there. He began to take up the reins of 'normal' living again.

Once Ed was back at home full time, attention turned to what to do about his teaching career. He wanted to return to his job (not least because he needed the money to cover his debts) and his head was prepared to accept him back, so a work hardening programme was implemented, with Ed attending the hospital as a day patient. First, he practised his teaching skills in a series of role-play teaching sessions (with volunteers from staff and other patients). The goals for one of his sessions were:

- To devise an accurate lesson plan.
- Describe clearly the concept of oxygen debt.
- Speak clearly and confidently.
- Have eye contact with everyone in the room.
- Answer questions appropriately.

His teaching ability proved to be excellent, but that only resolved part of the problem. He still had to return to the school, face his colleagues and, most importantly cope in the long term with the stress of his job. Through discussion it was decided that Ed should arrange a meeting at the school with the head teacher to consider the difficulties ahead. The head agreed that Ed could return to the school for 1 day a week initially, but that he should be supervised during all teaching sessions. Ed tried this out for a month and reviewed his progress in weekly follow-up sessions with the occupational therapist. The days themselves went fairly well, but at the end of the month Ed decided it was unrealistic to work as a teacher again. The treatment team concurred that this time it was probably the best decision, whilst recognising it was likely to have a negative impact on his prognosis.

Discussion

Ed's case highlights the ethical dilemma we often face, where our patient's interests may conflict with that of the wider society. Ed's therapist was strongly committed to helping him back to work, knowing it was his only remaining productive role and was important to him. But the therapist also recognised Ed was likely to become ill again and then what about the damage/disturbance he might cause to the school children and his colleagues? Furthermore the therapist was concerned for Ed that he was heading for another failure and that maybe it was time to cut his losses. In this particular case, Ed made his own decision not to return to work and the problem was somewhat bypassed. If you had been Ed's occupational therapist would you have been more active in encouraging him not to return to work?

Case illustration 7.6: Fran

Key issues   Behaviour and family problems, creative therapy

Summary of history

Fran, 15 years old, was admitted to an adolescent unit as a day patient. She had a history of behaviour problems and had been excluded from school after setting fire to a small class room. Her parents reported that she was out of their control with her rebellious, abusive behaviour. Some examples of her behaviour they gave were when she: smashed up the family crockery, was routinely aggressive to her siblings and came home drunk having stayed out all night. Fran's frequent arguments with her parents usually culminated in her locking herself in her room for hours, saying her parents did not understand her. Her behaviour at school was also problematic – her teachers described her as 'part of the deviant group who play truant and take drugs'. Fran herself admitted to smoking cannabis and trying Ecstacy on quite a few occasions.

Team strategy

The unit (which ran along therapeutic community lines) worked with Fran primarily using groupwork. The community functioned using general ward community meetings where the adolescents took 'control' of the meeting and were 'responsible' for each other. In addition a number of other set groups were held daily, which the residents were expected to attend. The three main types of groups offered were:

1. Psychotherapy groups (dramatherapy and small group verbal psychotherapy).
2. Life skills groups (social skills training and educational groups).
3. Work groups (woodwork, cooking or sports).

The team had a division of labour whereby the doctors and the social worker were responsible for family therapy; the doctors, occupational therapist and some senior nurses led the psychotherapy groups; and the nurses, teachers and occupational therapist ran the more practical groups.

Initial occupational therapy assessment

The first fortnight of Fran joining the community activities was designated as her assessment period (as opposed to formal one-to-one procedures). Specific assessment tools used within the groups included a projective art exercise of 'draw your family' and self-identity self-rating questionnaires. Key points from the assessment findings included:

1. *Feelings.* Fran showed herself to be angry and frustrated with her family and situation, whilst also being unhappy and uncertain about her own identity. She felt that her parents hated her and saw her as a failure. On her part, she wished they were not so old and lacking in understanding. Fran expressed feeling worthless except when she was with her friends and could 'have a good time'.
2. *Behaviour.* Fran found authority and assertion situations particularly difficult. In both, she escalated the situation and became aggressive/abusive. Her periodic 'acting out' behaviour indicated limited internal controls. She got on well with her peers though, as a leader, was occasionally inclined to bully others. On the other hand, she was skilled in many ways being quick thinking and creative, plus she had a bright sense of humour.

Treatment planning

Aims/objectives	Treatment methods
• To explore angry, ambivalent feelings about her parents. • To develop greater self-awareness and insight into what triggers behaviour. • To learn the differences between assertion and aggression. • To develop her self-esteem so she could see herself as a worthy person.	• Once-weekly dramatherapy session using mainly interaction games and role play. • Once weekly projective art. • Groupwork in general (including printing and magazine class) to highlight her strengths/assets and offer success experience.

Progress of treatment

Fran's stay at the day unit was an opportunity 'to grow' and 'time out' from the vicious cycle of negative experiences with which she was involved. She gained self-awareness and a more positive self-esteem from the community experiences.

In her projective art sessions Fran expressed a number of aggressive, destructive feelings (e.g. drawing herself as a monster for a painting titled 'what I am like inside'), but she also had the opportunity to explore what she liked about herself. This latter activity she initially found difficult to do, but gradually, after several similar activities, she was able to admit to positive things about herself.

In dramatherapy, Fran enjoyed the close groupwork and the fun of the lively games. Eventually she also came to share her feelings about her family. One significant activity for her was a family 'sculpt', looking at her family in the present and how she would like them to be in the future. This opened up several scenarios of how Fran could help bring the two images closer together. The regular family therapy sessions were also a significant growth point for Fran, with the opening up of generational communication and negotiating the giving of more positive things to each other.

Fran attended the day hospital full-time for 2 months and then 1 day a week for another 3 months whilst she returned to school. During this latter period much use was made of follow-up work and contracts to encourage her motivation to attend school and make it a constructive experience.

Discussion

In Fran's treatment, projective art was a central activity. The occupational therapist who used this medium drew on both psychodynamic and humanistic ideas. At the psychodynamic end of the spectrum the art was used as a means of tapping unconscious material and as a way of channelling aggressions (through projection). She was able to explore her boundaries and ambivalence about being so 'powerful'. On the humanistic side, Fran was encouraged to explore her self-concept (particularly the positive aspects) and exercise her creativity. Also the therapist never attempted to interpret Fran's pictures – preferring instead to ask Fran what she thought. In some ways the treatment stands in danger of being uncomfortably contradictory as the focus of the two approaches is different, with the psychodynamic approach centred on interpretations and past/unconscious material, and humanistic approach highlighting the spontaneous expressions of the here-and-now. However, in this case illustration the two approaches were able to coexist, as the therapist was primarily being humanistic. Most therapists will have their own aims and implicitly select one or other approach (e.g. projection = psychodynamic; self-awareness = humanistic).

Case illustration 7.7: Joe

Key issues   Senile dementia, assessment, reality orientation

Summary of history
Joe, a 70-year-old bachelor, was admitted to an assessment unit for elderly people, with a diagnosis of senile dementia. Whilst being physically healthy, he had a 1 year history of increasing forgetfulness and being unsafe at home. His neighbours and the social worker reported that he has frequently wandered or got lost while out shopping. The warden in his warden-controlled flat reported he was often unsafe (i.e. he often left the gas on). She also commented that Joe was socially isolated except for regular contacts with his home help.

Team strategy
The nurses and the occupational therapist were the key people involved in assessing Joe's functioning to consider whether to return him home or to apply for Part III accommodation. The ward also operated a continuous reality orientation programme and, as such, the team's approach to Joe needs to be consistent, reinforcing relevant information such as where he was and the time of day. The nursing staff played a key role in Joe's daily management, whilst the occupational therapist ran a range of activity groups.

Initial occupational therapy assessment
Assessment was carried out using the standardised CAPE assessment plus general observation in tasks and activity sessions on the ward. The findings can be summarised as:

1. *Behaviour.* Joe presented as having a well-preserved personality, being friendly, with a sense of humour, and looking clean and tidy. He was able to interact politely with others, but he found carrying out a conversation difficult (see below).
2. *Cognitive.* Joe was disorientated in time and place. His recent recall was impaired but he had a fair long-term memory. In tasks he got confused when using tools and was easily distracted having poor concentration (less than 5 minutes). Joe exhibited some expressive and receptive language difficulties and he found it easier to respond to visual cues than answer direct questions.
3. *Feelings.* Occasionally Joe became aggressive, or indicated that he was frus-

trated and lacking in confidence. This occurred particularly at the times when he had insight into his problems. Mostly, however, Joe remained cheerful and open to having some 'gentlemanly fun'.

Treatment planning

Aims/objectives	Treatment methods
• With a view to returning to his flat, assess safety and ability in: using the gas fire, making tea, and using the intercom (as required for his particular complex). With a view to Part III, ensure independence in mobility and self-care.	Practical assessments using appropriate tools.
• During hospital stay attempt to reduce confusion and maintain or improve orientation and memory.	Staff approach (e.g. reinforcing main information) and encouraging him to keep a notebook handy to refer to regularly.
• Maintain/improve task performance skills.	Two daily activity sessions involving familiar crafts, card games, dominoes and light physical exercise.
• Provide social involvements.	Use of group/social activities, especially dance and music.
• Activate long-term memories and stimulate more recent recollections.	Reminiscence therapy using photographs, music and limited discussion, ensuring present-day orientation.
• Maintain dignity and sense of individuality by giving him productive roles.	Put Joe in charge of watering plants, including two of his own special ones brought from home; staff approach also important.

Progress of treatment

After a month-long admission, the team recommended Joe be referred for Part III accommodation as his cognitive difficulties made him unsafe for independent living and it was felt he was likely to deteriorate further. Joe returned to his flat, whilst his waiting list place came through. For the most part he seemed to enjoy the social contact and stimulation in the unit. On his discharge a slight improvement in his social ability was noted prompting the team to advise him to try to develop more social contacts.

Discussion

Joe's case illustrates two problems/dilemmas which frequently confront us in our working life.

First, we often deal with long-term, continuing handicaps where deterioration is a constant reality against which we battle. Our aims of treatment revolve around maintaining function rather than improving it. For some therapists this can seem an unsatisfying, waste of time and resources. For others it is exciting work, made meaningful by achieving realistic, small objectives and the feeling of performing a worthwhile job.

Secondly, Joe's case reminds us that the realities of scarce resources mean we sometimes have to settle for less than ideal solutions. The treatment team were reluctant to discharge Joe home as there were clear risks to his safety. However, the assessment unit was unable to hold patients for longer than a month and there was no other suitable facility available for Joe to use whilst waiting for his new accommodation.

Case illustration 7.8: Phillip

Key issues   Inadequate personality disorder and practical goal setting

Summary of history

Phillip, 21 years old, was admitted to an acute unit having attempted suicide with an aspirin overdose. He did not know why he had done this, except that he felt confused and uncertain about his future, having just completed his university degree. On more detailed assessment it was discovered that he had a distant relationship with his parents who led active business and social lives but a close relationship with their live-in housekeeper. Having spent his first year of university in a hall of residence, Phillip had moved back to live at home, where his food/laundry needs were supplied.

Team strategy

The psychiatrist saw Phillip for individual psychotherapy and (with the social worker) for a few family therapy meetings. It was decided that the occupational therapist should help Phillip with his practical coping skills.

Initial occupational therapy assessment

Phillip presented as being passive, lacking initiative and dependent on others. On interview, using OCAIRS, he expressed feeling he 'should be man enough' to live independently, but felt unable to do so. He did not know what he wanted to do in the future and felt he had little control over it (except that he agreed he wanted to live rather than to die). His degree was a good one, but in life he felt a failure. A practical group cooking session showed Phillip's skills to be limited to egg-on-toast, though he enjoyed the experience of both working in a group and producing a lunch. Use of the Interest Checklist demonstrated that Phillip had a mild interest in art, cooking and stamp collecting but he had not pursued any hobby seriously.

Treatment planning

Aims/objectives	Treatment methods
1. To develop practical and domestic independence skills and to experience confidence in self as an effective, competent and independent person.	(a) Regular cooking group sessions to learn and practise skills. (b) Attendance once-weekly at 'life skills' group –

<table>
<tr><td></td><td>encompassing discussion, support and practical tasks.</td></tr>
<tr><td>2. To develop a sense of agency and personal responsibility; and to explore (realistic) options for the future regarding jobs, living independently, developing social contacts, etc.</td><td>Once-weekly one-to-one client-centred counselling session to set goals and consider different life options.</td></tr>
</table>

Progress of treatment

The key to Phillip's long-term treatment was the practical goal setting (behavioural strategy) which he negotiated weekly with the occupational therapist (using a client-centred approach). He found that having a goal in written form helped to make it a concrete realistic possibility, and also having to 'feedback' the results, ensured he fulfilled the goal. Some examples of goals he attempted latterly included:

1. Visit one specific art exhibition of choice.
2. Investigate possible day/night classes on offer in the area.
3. Sign up with the local cookery course and make arrangements for attendance.
4. Cook a complete meal for the family.
5. Investigate possible places to live for the future, comparing options, prices and viability, prior to discussion in the 'life skills' group.

Phillip was discharged as an in-patient after a fortnight, but continued to attend sessions as a out-patient. He eventually found his own place to live (whilst maintaining social contacts with his family) and was beginning to look for a job when he was discharged.

Discussion

Phillip's treatment was largely focused on developing practical, independence skills. Treatment could equally have been targeted towards Phillip's work role. In this case, the therapist reasoned (by employing narrative, interactive and pragmatic clinical reasoning) it would be unhelpful to focus on work as he may well have been unable to get a job at the end of treatment. By helping Phillip become more skilled, purposeful and confident, the therapist hoped his long-term employment chances would be improved. Was the therapist being unduly pessimistic or realistic? It is never easy to decide treatment priorities as there are many factors to consider. This therapist was at least responsible enough to weigh up different treatment options with him, rather than simply assume a desired course.

Case illustration 7.9: Kevin

Key issues   Development of play skills and play therapy

Summary of history

Kevin, an 8-year-old boy, was referred to a child and family psychiatry day unit after being suspended from school for his antisocial behaviour. He had a history of behaviour problems and bullying other children. Kevin was seen to have a close relationship with his mother who tended to overprotect and cosset him, occasionally limiting his social contact with other children. This was due, in part, to Kevin's history of epilepsy, though largely controlled now with medication.

Team strategy

Each team member had a specific role to play: the nurses and unit teachers worked on Kevin's social interaction/behaviour; the psychologist investigated his cognitive functioning; the social worker engaged the parents in family therapy; the doctors reviewed the medication and took an overall management role; and the occupational therapist acted as a play therapist.

Initial occupational therapy assessment

The occupational therapist initially attempted to use non-directive play with Kevin, offering 'free play' and a non-judgmental approach. This proved unworkable, however, as Kevin seemed unable to play and resorted to requesting structured, competitive board games. The occupational therapist decided to work more directively using play. Through puppets, painting and dressing-up activities, Kevin revealed his lack of imaginative/fantasy play (i.e. developmentally he seems to have missed out the play stage between 3 and 7 years). Further, when uncertain about what to do next, he often became aggressive or demanded to play a competitive game saying 'I'm going to win!' The occupational therapist hypothesised that a key problem for Kevin was his limited play skills, which in turn severely affected his peer interactions. On the strength side, he was bright, with many other abilities (e.g. school work) and also he wanted to make friends with others (though had never been able to do so).

Treatment planning

Aims/objectives	Treatment methods
1. Establish a relationship with Kevin (making it 'safe' for him to lose occasionally as well as boosting his esteem).	Twice-weekly individual sessions with the occupational therapist taking a positive and encouraging attitude, whilst confronting him about his difficulties.
2. Teach how to 'play' – encouraging flexibility, having fun and using imagination.	Grade each activity for its imagination level, acting first as a model.
3. Lessen intensity for winning competitive games.	Discuss issues of winning and losing, trying to practise handling the latter.

Progress of treatment

First, a contract was established whereby Kevin could choose any activity he wanted to do for the last 10 minutes of the session, providing he joined in the occupational therapist's set activities earlier. The therapist invented a structured, competitive game which eventually could act as fantasy play. On trying to work constructively with Kevin's aggression, she devised a competition of 'knocking down toy soldiers in the sandpit by throwing small plastic balls'. Kevin enjoyed this and it became his 'choice game' as well. The therapist approached the game encouraging the fun element, by using laughter and playing little games within, like 'throwing all the balls in one go, really quickly'. When the intensity for winning was reduced in Kevin and he simply enjoyed his sessions, the occupational therapist increasingly added the element of imagination, e.g. speculating on what a soldier was thinking or felt like. The natural progression became more focus on the sandpit playing with the soldiers, having them fight and help each other, building barriers, inventing scenarios, etc. When Kevin was thoroughly familiar with this play other children were invited in for short periods to join in 'Kevin's game' which they all found great fun.

Discussion

Kevin's treatment lies within a developmental framework of teaching skills. In common with all treatments we offer, alternative methods based on other theoretical frameworks are possible. Kevin's problem may well have been seen as a behavioural one with his aggression to peers being targeted as the priority area for treatment (the problem which the nurse prioritised). Here, behaviour modification using star charts and modelling could have been incorporated into a group activities programme. The humanistic occupational therapist, following the Axline approach, may have diagnosed an unhappy, lonely child, who needed to explore his feelings within an accepting relationship. The decision of which approach to take was largely organised according to the team's negotiation in an attempt to balance interventions. To some extent trial-and-error also had a part to play (e.g. the initial unsuccessful use of free play).

Case illustration 7.10: Mrs Brown

Key issues   Bereavement, family and community support

Summary of history

Mrs Brown, a 76-year-old widow, had deteriorated markedly over the previous year since the death of her husband. She had neglected herself physically, being both depressed and forgetful. Living alone, she had become increasingly dependent on her married daughter who lived nearby. The daughter was concerned about her mother's poor self-care, safety and isolation, and had sought help from the general practitioner.

Team strategy

The general practitioner did a preliminary assessment on Mrs Brown and referred her to the Community Mental Health Team. On discussion, they decided that the occupational therapist should become the key worker, given her skills in both practical assessments and counselling, using back-up services as necessary (e.g. social worker to organise financial aspects and practical services). The team was concerned to assess Mrs Brown's exact level of functioning in her home and to consider the future possibilities.

Initial occupational therapy assessment

Two home visits were undertaken. The first aimed at establishing initial contact with Mrs Brown and her daughter, the second focused on Mrs Brown individually. Methods used were interview and observation using the task of making soup and a cup of tea. Key findings included:

1. *Skills*. She was physically slow and absent-minded when making tea, looked slightly dishevelled in her self-care and tended to neglect feeding herself.
2. *Feelings*. She became tearful when talking about husband and said she did not want to do anything except sit.
3. *Behaviour*. She was dependent on her daughter and was less capable/more feeble when daughter was around.
4. *Social*. She was isolated and had little social contact except for her daughter's input.

The positive aspects identified included:

1. The fact that Mrs Brown's activities of daily living skills seem safe and intact, providing she concentrated on the task.
2. The daughter's willingness to be supportive.
3. The comfortable semi-detached bungalow which Mrs Brown owns and loves.

Treatment planning

Aims/objectives	Treatment methods
1. To gain emotional support (considering her self-neglect within this).	Two days a week at the day unit offering: (a) Craft groups for social aspects. (b) Cooking group to assess practical
2. Further assess domestic/self-care skills to ensure safety.	skills. (c) Individual support/bereavement counselling.
3. Explore mother–daughter relationship and how they manage practically.	Two joint sessions to negotiate mutual roles and time given by daughter, considering their individual needs.
4. To engage in hobby interests and pursue opportunities for social contact.	Encourage Mrs Brown to join social clubs, evening classes or do some voluntary work.

Progress of treatment

Mrs Brown was initially reluctant to go to the day unit, feeling both apathetic and uncertain about new life changes. She was persuaded to go for a trial period when her daughter agreed to drop and collect her by car. Once she settled into the day unit she enjoyed the social contact and re-learned some old craft hobbies. The occupational therapist also saw Mrs Brown regularly on a one-to-one basis, offering support and allowing her to express feelings of her loss.

The cooking sessions exposed some potential problems as Mrs Brown was occasionally unsafe, remaining slightly forgetful and confused – in any case, she was not motivated to cook for herself. The issue of Mrs Brown's potential self-neglect regarding feeding herself, and her daughter's subsequent 'over-involve-ment', became the focus of treatment. A contract was established where Mrs Brown received lunch via meals-on-wheels (WRVS) or the day hospital, and she provided her own cold breakfast and evening snacks. Instead of cooking regularly for her mother the daughter was encouraged to invite Mrs Brown to Sunday lunch with family.

In the long term, Mrs Brown enjoyed going regularly to an activities centre for the over 60s. The occupational therapist continued to monitor her situation by vis-iting every few months over a period of 1 year.

Discussion
A number of questions are raised about the role adopted by this occupational therapist. The occupational therapist here mainly adopted a counselling role, whilst the practical craft and cooking sessions at the day hospital were run by an occupational therapy helper. It could be argued that the occupational therapist was not really doing 'occupational therapy', except at a management level supervising the helper. As this is a fairly common scenario, I would suggest it is an acceptable role for occupational therapists. More so because the occupational therapist main-tained a focus on Mrs Brown's occupational performance, i.e. she did not get side tracked into being a bereavement counsellor.

However, the therapist did become involved in offering some individual bereavement counselling, which raises questions as she did not have any specific counselling training. Whilst acknowledging it would have been difficult (and unrealistic) not to get involved in doing some supportive work related to Mrs Brown's bereavement, she might have been better advised to recommend Mrs Brown see a trained counsellor or perhaps refer her on to a relevant organisation such as CRUSE. What do you think?

Case illustration 7.11: Roy

Key issues   Acute psychotic episode and 'Directive Group Therapy'

Summary of history
Roy, a 30-year-old man, was admitted to hospital with a diagnosis of schizophre-nia, having been found by the police wandering through traffic and threatening passers by. On admission he was thought disordered, paranoid, aggressive and his behaviour was bizarre as he responded to 'voices'. Roy had a long history of suf-fering from acute episodes and chronic negative symptoms (poor motivation, flat-tening of affect and social withdrawal). Six months previously, he had been discharged from a secure unit where he had been detained for over 2 years for his violent behaviour. Since that time he has been socially isolated, unemployed and often lived rough. His florid symptoms recurred when he stopped taking his med-ication.

Team strategy
The initial priority for the treatment team (at this stage the nurses and doctors) was to get Roy re-stabilised on medication and to contain his behaviour. After a month

of admission the team thought Roy was sufficiently stable for some occupational therapy input to prepare him for his transfer onto a long-term rehabilitation ward.

Initial occupational therapy assessment

Using a combination of assessments (such as the AOF and Volitional Questionnaire) the occupational therapist summarised her findings:

- *Volition.* (a) Some interest shown in dominoes and art; (b) if prompted/directed Roy will join in structured activities; (c) passive and hypoactive (in part due to sedating affects of medication).
- *Habituation.* (a) Has no productive roles; (b) institutionalised passive behaviour; does not initiate action; (c) requires structure and routine.
- *Performance.* (a) Task performance skills poor: follows basic one step instructions; poor concentration and motivation which interferes with task completion; motor skills within normal limits. (b) Social behaviour: poor social skills; unresponsive and difficult to interact with; suspicious of others and tends to stare at them.

Treatment planning

Aims/objectives	Treatment methods
1. To engage in productive role behaviour. 2. To maintain and develop task performance skills in particular develop concentration and task completion. 3. To maintain and develop appropriate social interaction (eye contact, co-operation and basic conversation skills).	Using the model of human occupation as a framework for treatment: 'Directive Group Therapy' (Kaplan, 1986) – a daily group lasting for 1 hour carrying out a range of practical activities; e.g. art and cooking.

Progress of treatment

Roy attended the Directive Group daily (sometimes he needed to be brought down by a nurse) for several weeks. The group provided a vital daily structure and routine for Roy to maintain and develop basic functional skills. He became slightly more responsive in his social behaviour – though his 'staring' remained a problem and others continued to feel threatened in his presence. His concentration improved significantly such that he was able to attend to and complete tasks over the course of the hour long group. Roy responded best whilst playing dominoes which he enjoyed. He also proved to be adept at being a 'creative curry cook' – a skill he learned from his grandmother.

The group was of particular value as it provided a point of continuity for Roy when he was transferred on to the rehabilitation ward. The nurses on the rehabilitation ward took over responsibility for his domestic rehabilitation. For the long term, the team aimed to refer Roy to a day centre with a CPN involved to ensure Roy kept up his medication.

Discussion

This case illustration reminds me that sometimes the treatment team has to accept less than ideal outcomes. Some problems may be too complex, too deep or out of our control and we can do little about them. However, that does not diminish the value of what we *can* offer.

Roy's treatment team needed to take care that they were realistic in their expectations for his long-term future. His prognosis was fairly poor. He was likely to remain socially isolated and was unlikely ever to be employed. He was also going to need continuous long-term support to monitor his mental state/ensure he kept up with his medication and to provide him with appropriate day care for social contact. Of course such long-term support carries resourcing implications (namely availability of day centre places and long-term CPN cover) which cannot be taken for granted and could present problems in the future. With adequate community support and follow-up, however, the team could be hopeful that Roy's condition would be positively managed. Arguably, this type of long-term 'disability management' (Richards, 1996) should be our main occupational therapy aim.

Case illustration 7.12: Marge

Key issues   Manic depression, domestic role, time structuring

Summary of history

Marge, 40 years old, was referred to the local day hospital for treatment with a diagnosis of bipolar affective disorder (manic depression). Recently she had been in a depressed phase where she simply lay in bed all day. This culminated in her taking an overdose of sleeping pills (but her husband discovered her in time). On other occasions Marge has been excessively active, doing domestic chores around the house, showing a difficulty in pacing herself and activities, which has resulted in her collapsing at the end of the day. Marge was first diagnosed as having manic depression 10 years previously, when she had been under a considerable amount of stress from looking after her active twin daughters. The twins left home last year, but she has kept up cleaning their room regularly. Now she has the added stress of caring for a demanding invalid father-in-law who has come to live with them. Marge has had a strained relationship with her husband, exacerbated by his redundancy from work which has resulted in him being at home all day.

Team strategy

The team's overall strategy is to ensure Marge's extreme mood swings are largely controlled by medication and monitored long term by the doctors. The social worker was asked to become involved in doing some marital work. The team agreed that the occupational therapist should help Marge with her role at home and daily time structuring.

Initial occupational therapy assessment

Marge was assessed over a couple of weeks using a range of tools, e.g. Interview (using OPHI), Activity Record, Interest checklist, cooking task-group, home visit. The following interlinked problems were identified:

1. Difficulty in planning realistic (and balanced) daily timetable.
2. Lack of acceptance of daughters leaving home with the attached implications of her reduced domestic/mother role.
3. Habits and mental set of caring for others to the point of exhaustion, rather than giving space for herself.
4. Lack of social contacts or interests/hobbies outside of domestic role and family.

On her strength side, she showed much ability and knowledge of houseworking skills, and was basically kind and helpful to others. She also receives some emotional and social support from her family.

Treatment planning

Aims/objectives	Treatment methods
• To develop the ability to plan a realistic and balanced timetable (aiming to continue such a routine in the long term).	Daily timetable and weekly activities programme to be regularly negotiated with therapist.
• To learn to negotiate an acceptable domestic division of labour with her husband.	Planned with support of the therapist and social worker in the marital sessions.
• To experience an increase in her self-esteem; to feel valued and able.	Involvement in a range of activities/groups offering success experiences, new relationships, e.g. relaxation and dance, and helping 'co-run' the cookery group.
• To develop a hobby interest which can be pursued in the long term	Dressmaking class (her choice)

Progress of treatment

Marge was initially uncertain and lacking in confidence in dressmaking, but it soon developed into an exciting project for her where she became involved with fabric printing as well as making clothes for herself and her family. She pursued her interest by joining a local dressmaking class which further developed her skills and offered her a new social outlet.

Marge's timetabling skills remained problematic and she continued to need prompting to contain her activities and help maintain a balanced programme. This role was eventually taken over by her husband who also participated by planning a more constructive programme for himself. He was also more supportive in helping out with domestic tasks.

Marge was discharged from the day hospital after a few months. She seemed happier and more confident with her fuller life and skills though she remained somewhat vulnerable to her mood swings. She had so enjoyed her time at the day hospital and participating in the activities, that she eventually joined the 'ex-patients' activities club', which met once a week.

Discussion

This case example highlights a common aspects of much of our work in the mental health field. We deal with serious psychiatric illnesses, where the prognosis regarding relapse ranges from fair to poor which may make us question the value of our treatment. At these times we need to return to the idea that we do not treat a diagnosis but instead attempt to help a person cope better in their daily lives. Hopefully, our choice of priority problems to tackle will have a relevant impact on the person's future capacity to cope. In Marge's case, the occupational therapist was not in a position to do much about the illness of manic depression; nor was the occupational therapist able to take away Marge's life stresses, such as being a carer. Treatment instead, had to have a more limited (but valuable) aim, i.e. namely helping Marge manage her time and occupational behaviour better.

CONCLUSION

Having considered the case illustrations in this chapter, what kind of conclusions can be drawn about our occupational therapy role and practice? Here are my thoughts.

Focus on occupations and activities

All of the examples showed the occupational therapist focusing on peoples' daily occupations and their occupational performance. Also, activities were used therapeutically in some way with all the patients/clients. Although some therapists might favour a 'counselling' approach (as Catherine's therapist did), the emphasis of therapy can still be encouraging the person to be active – the thrust of treatment is 'doing'.

Eclectic theoretical base

We employ a wide range of theoretical frameworks – using both occupational therapy models (as shown with Roy's treatment) and psychological approaches (e.g. psychodynamic methods with Fran and the behavioural methods with George). We also pragmatically integrate different models and approaches (as seen in Sally's treatment).

Multiple assessment methods

We also employ a wide range of assessment methods – both informal (Mrs Brown's interview) and formal (the use of standardised assessments in Steve's treatment). Often occupational therapists will use a combination of several assessments (such as the battery given to Marge).

Community focus

Most of the examples demonstrated our bias towards looking at a person's functioning and daily life roles in the community. Even when we work in acute hospital settings, our focus is usually on the person's longer-term functioning (Roy's treatment was an exception here) and we often act as a bridge between hospital and community.

Teamwork

In some of the examples occupational therapy played a central role (e.g. being Mrs Brown's key worker), whilst with others the occupational therapist was a more marginal contributor (such as with Kevin and Roy). Our role must always be taken in the context of the overall team strategy. It is only by working in a team that we can hope to make treatment 'holistic'. How can one professional ever hope to do everything?!

8   Evaluation

Our integrity and confidence as therapists is derived from our ability to evaluate what we do and as such it must be a central component of our practice. Evaluation is often considered to be the last stage of the occupational therapy process coming after identifying problems and implementing treatment. In reality, it is much more than this. We evaluate continuously throughout treatment in order to ensure what we are doing is effective. Often treatment does not progress in the anticipated or desired manner and new problems may emerge which require attention (see Theory into Practice box below). We also evaluate to safeguard good standards of occupational therapy practice in our service. This applies throughout our professional development and constitutes our quality assurance.

What is involved in evaluation? Broadly speaking we can divide evaluation into: (a) evaluation of the treatment process and (b) research, which is a longer term evaluation. This chapter aims to show how both of these areas have a critical role to play in the development of occupational therapy services and our profession as a whole.

THEORY INTO PRACTICE

The need for on-going evaluation

Ben's situation is a good example of rehabilitation that lacked sufficient evaluation of a kind which might have pre-empted further 'mistakes'.

Problem situation
Ben is a 26-year-old man with a learning disability. He was brought up by his mother, living at home and attending a day centre. He functioned well and fairly independently until his mother died 2 years ago. Ben was taken into the local institution for shelter and with a view to rehabilitation and resettlement. After some initial 'behaviour problems', Ben settled down to the new routines of living in a supervised half-way house and working in the local sheltered work unit. He was well liked, skilled and reliable in his work. After some preparation, when places

came up, he was discharged to a group home in the community. Two weeks later Ben returned to hospital in a state of anxiety and exhibiting a range of behaviour problems.

Analysis

The treatment team carefully evaluated Ben's current situation, recognising the following problem areas:

1. Problems with Ben: anxiety; behaviour problems; sense of failure; lack of confidence; fear of the future; issues of bereavement and loss resurfaced.
2. Problems within his environment: group home residents not operating as a supportive, co-operative unit; workshop fairly pressured, with an impatient, authoritarian manager.
3. Inadequate treatment: treatment process was too quick/not graded carefully enough with visits, overnight stays, etc.; too many changes pushed through at once; not enough attention given to bereavement aspects of terminating hospital stay; inadequate liaison with workshop manager; inadequate follow-up support.

Problem-solving plan

In the initial stages, allow Ben the sanctuary of hospital to rebuild confidence and gain support. Gradually resettle into a group home in the middle stages, maintaining active support. He should continue working in the sheltered workshop within the hospital for security.

8.1 EVALUATING THE TREATMENT PROCESS

It is our professional responsibility to evaluate the treatment process and our occupational therapy practice. This evaluation needs to occur at different levels. We need to review patient's/client's progress and monitor the effectiveness of the treatment as a whole. At a broader level we are also being asked, increasingly, to evaluate the quality of our service provision (via clinical audit). Finally, we need to evaluate ourselves as therapists. This section will review these four areas and describe the range of both objective and subjective tools in current use.

Evaluating patient's/client's progress

There are a number of ways to assess the progress of a patient/client in treatment. At the most basic level we can ask our patients/clients if they feel any progress. Sometimes when dealing with mental health problems it is difficult to pinpoint exactly what has changed, but the person, somehow, 'feels' better. As well as eliciting their view we can record any tangible progress that has taken place. For instance, the person might smile more and show more spontaneity or enthusiasm to engage in activity.

Beyond these informal and fairly subjective ways of monitoring progress we can (and arguably should) use more objective measures (e.g. **outcome measures**).

Outcome measures involve measuring systematically, the results or outcomes of treatment by comparing measurements to either pre-treatment objectives or assessment results. Three different types of measures (objectives, functional and subjective) are distinguished below.

Objectives as outcome measures

One way of measuring a patient's/client's progress is to compare what has been achieved against the objectives set. Thus, the objective becomes the criteria for identifying effectiveness of treatment. For example, consider the following objective: 'At the end of 2 weeks treatment Malcolm should be able to follow written instructions for a basic woodwork task, independently. Here the *criteria* for successful achievement is clearly stated so offers a clear outcome measure. Vague aims of treatment such as 'improve task performance' cannot act as an outcome measure and are thus less helpful for pinpointing progress.

THEORY INTO PRACTICE

Evaluating why patients/clients have not met objectives

There are a number of reasons why, on evaluation, we may find a patient/client has not progressed or achieved desired objectives. To investigate why, we should start by asking whether or not the original objectives were appropriate and realistic. If the answer is 'yes', then we would look for alternative explanations, i.e.

1. Factors located within the *individual*. For instance, he or she may have relapsed and the symptoms of the illness may be interfering with functioning; equally the individual may have improved markedly, rendering the treatment inappropriate; alternatively he or she may be lack motivation (perhaps as a result of lack of stimulation in the environment).
2. Factors concerning the person's *environment*. Family members may be resisting treatment; alternatively contradictory staff attitudes or hostile community reactions may be proving destructive.
3. Factors related to *team treatment*. The treatment team need to take some responsibility if treatment is not producing desired results. Here, we might look out for poor initial assessment, poor timing of interventions, too much stimulation/challenge, inadequate grading, lack of team co-operation, etc.

Functional measures

Functional measures offer a way of measuring improvement in a person's functioning before, during and after treatment. Ideally standardised assessments should be used as they (technically) result in more valid/reliable scores which can then be used as a basis for comparison (see the Theory into Practice below).

THEORY INTO PRACTICE

Two standardised tests yielding functional measures

CAPE (Clifton Assessment Procedures for the Elderly)
This test aims to assess cognitive and behavioural competence related to levels of dependency in elderly people. As one example, consider the use of the Behaviour Rating Scale which asks the 'carer' 18 questions about the elderly individual, such as:

He/she keeps him/herself occupied in a constructive or useful activity (works, reads, plays games, has hobbies, etc.):

almost always occupied	0
sometimes occupied	1
almost never occupied	2

Clearly, if before treatment the carer's responses totalled 20 (for the 18 items) and went down to 10 after treatment, we have a clear-cut measure of improvement (i.e. the person went from being in the 'maximum' to 'medium dependency band').

Barthel ADL Scale
The Barthel is a well used standardised ADL scale which aims to measure independence in personal care. It covers 10 items including feeding, transfers, grooming/hygiene, etc. Items are scored on a scale of 1–10 (with five being given for assisted performance and 10 implying maximum independence). Again the numerical score (say of 50 moving up to 80) offers a straightforward measure of improvements in functional performance.

Increasingly, research published in journals attests the benefits of different treatments and activities having measured improvement using particular tests. Take for example the study described by Moore and Bracegirdle (1994). They evaluated the effect of a 6-week exercise programme on feelings of well-being and happiness experienced by 15 elderly women by comparing their responses to a control group. The researchers utilised the Memorial University of Newfoundland Scale of Happiness (MUNSH) to measure any pre- and post-therapy improvements and concluded that exercise did indeed have a beneficial effect.

Subjective measures

Subjective measures aim to offer a way of measuring an individual's own perception of progress. Most self-rating assessments could be used here, though to maximise reliability and validity, published and well researched tools are recommended. The COPM (Canadian Occupational Performance Measure) is one such tool where clients identify their own needs and difficulties in occupational performance. For example, the client might identify 'active recreation such as outings and travel' as their most important problem which they rate on a scale of 1–10 for both performance and satisfaction. This offers a relatively clear-cut baseline from which to compare future scores (assuming the client uses a similar criteria the next time).

Evaluating the use of measures

So far, I have presented evaluation through outcome measures as an unproblematic process. The reality is not so straightforward!

First, measuring progress using objectives depends largely on how good the objectives were in the first place. For a start, it is possible to set trivial and easily achieved objectives to 'show' improvement – but these may not say anything abut the individual's overall progress.

Secondly, measuring improvement using standardised assessment scores is not infallible. We need to remember that no standardised assessment is completely valid and reliable. For one thing, the individual (or therapist) may perform in an uncharacteristic way during the test which biases the result (e.g. if they know what response is being sought); for another thing, the scores still have to be interpreted.

Thirdly, the use of functional measures using activities of daily living assessments have been hotly debated. Often they are limited in what they measure (for instance just personal ADL) so the extent to which they predict how well a person 'copes and feels' in their wider life can be questioned. Also some therapists feel their focus on practical functioning makes them less relevant in some mental health settings. For a wider discussion of their problems, see Eakin (1989a,b) and Hagedorn (1995).

Lastly, the use of subjective measures remains problematic as they lack controls for reliability (for instance individuals may score themselves differently from day to day depending on how they feel rather than on their objective performance). On the other hand, it could be argued that these measures have the most 'validity' and relevance if we are to be truly client-centred.

Evaluating treatment

Observation and analysis

Alongside the evaluation of progress using outcome measures we employ observation and analysis to evaluate treatment as a whole. To illustrate how this works in practice consider the three examples below. Examples 8.1 and 8.2 offer two different approaches to recording and evaluating the same group treatment session; example 8.3 illustrates a therapist's evaluation of the evolution of a group.

Example 8.1: Therapist's analysis and notes of a cooking group

The cooking group was initially tense as Karen vetoed everyone's suggestions. Eventually she agreed to spaghetti bolognese and apple crumble. Mario was elected as 'chief chef' as he had a special family recipe. He asked Bill to chop the vegetables and Sam and Kim to make the dessert. Karen stormed out saying there wasn't any point in her being there. Mario followed her to encourage her back to do the actual cooking.

Karen returned to cook the sauce and the group mood lifted. Karen flirted with Mario whilst he reminisced about his childhood in Italy. Bill was quiet but seemed to enjoy listening. Sam and Kim worked independently and well at the other cooker, though they isolated themselves from the group conversation.

Group evaluation: The meal worked well in the end and the group was productive. I facilitated some discussion about the group process suggesting that the sense of group/group spirit was still lacking. We discussed their individual roles, for instance that Mario was a positive leader and Bill a positive contributor whilst Karen remained self-absorbed. Karen acknowledged that she became attention seeking if she didn't get her own way. Sam and Kim understood their close, supportive relationship was potentially destructive to the rest of the group. See Figure 8.1.

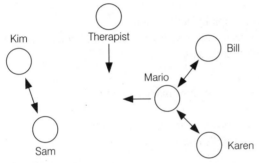

Figure 8.1 Sociogram of interactions.

Example 8.2: Using a 'group process' evaluation form
A. Group goals
  1. No goals
  ②Some goals or goals slightly confused
  3. Goals very clear
  Comments: *members tend to forget the group interaction goal and focus on the* task

B. Quantity/quality of work accomplished
  1. No work accomplished
  2. Average accomplishments
  ③Great deal of quality work accomplished
  Comments: *good lunch produced*

C. Group atmosphere
  ①Hostile, uncomfortable, negative
  ②Average, reasonable
  3. Highly supportive, co-operative, warm

Comments: *initially uncomfortable when Karen blocked suggestions, then ran out upset*

D. Group cohesion/trust
   1. Group fragmented or lacking in trust
   ②Average
   3. Strong sense of belonging and trust

E. Participation Comments: *group split into sub-groups*
   1. Limited and uneven
   ②Average
   3. Great deal of group member involvement
   Comments: *Mario needed to encourage and support Karen to keep her in the group; Bill largely silent but encouraging*

F. Sensitivity
   1. Group members self-absorbed, insensitive
   ②Average
   3. Outstanding empathy and listening
   Comments: *Karen self-absorbed; Sam and Kim isolated; Mario shows good empathy and facilitating skill*

G. Group decisions
   ①No decisions or decisions made by a few
   2. Majority decisions accepted
   3. Full participation and consensus achieved
   Comments: *eventually consensus achieved*

Example 8.3: Therapist's analysis of a psychotherapy group's evolving themes
Early stage – Forming and norming themes:
   (a) reactions to therapists; questioning their authority/status/ability; testing them
   (b) sharing 'secrets'; coming out; recognising commonality of experience
   (c) denial of anger (against parents, medical system)

Middle stage – Norming and performing themes:
   (a) bingeing on emotions – members expressing/exploring many feelings
   (b) high identification, support and sharing between members
   (c) competition with siblings acknowledged related to negative self-image

Late stage – Storming and performing themes:
   (a) transferences onto therapists explored especially anger with 'mother'
   (b) individual stories explored (e.g. P's experience of being abused)
   (c) issues of future coping explored

Ending stage – Storming and performing themes:
   (a) resistance to group ending explored
   (b) recognition of the link between unexpressed emotion and eating disorder
   (c) future goals stated

All of these examples above show the therapist as actively observing, reasoning, analysing and evaluating treatment. Rather than being done mentally, information like this should be recorded in writing. This ensures a more disciplined analysis plus is open to wider public scrutiny. Furthermore having proper records offers a baseline for future evaluation.

User feedback

Arguably, any evaluation must take into account the patient's/client's own view of their treatment. After all, they are the ones to use the service and we need to be responsive to their experiences.

There are a number of structured methods we can use to gain feedback including:

1. *Verbal feedback at the end of a treatment.* Individual or group members share (e.g. verbally) 'one thing he or she found difficult' and 'one thing gained'.
2. *Use of an evaluation form.* One variety of evaluation form is the type that is given out after a groupwork course (e.g. a questionnaire about an anxiety management course and asking how helpful it has been).
3. *Consumer questionnaire.* It might be desirable to design a consumer questionnaire as part of clinical audit, researching how well the service is meeting patients'/clients' needs. Questions could ask for information about how quickly they were seen; how clear they were about aims of treatment; if they had any complaints and how they were dealt with, etc.

Service evaluation and clinical audit

Clinical audit is a systematic process undertaken to ensure the quality of treatment interventions or, more generally, of the service provided (sometimes called service audit). As purchasers and health care policy makers demand evidence that treatment is effective (related to efficacy and cost effectiveness), clinical audit is becoming a necessary part of managing a service. Increasingly we are being asked to specify the value of what we do and we are questioned if the best outcome has been achieved for the least cost. As Foto (1996) notes, 'It is no longer enough for us to simply say that a patient got better. We have to develop measures that clearly define what better is ...' (p. 87).

Audit starts with asking certain question about the service, namely concerning its:

1. *Structure* (e.g. staff training, physical resources, lines of communication, numbers of patients treated).
2. *Process* (e.g. referral system, assessment and treatment techniques).
3. *Outcome* (e.g. whether or not treatment objectives have been met).

The kinds of questions we might want to answer in a clinical audit relate to four issues:

- *Quality*. Are the clinical services offered appropriate for meeting the needs of local people? How long do patients have to wait between being referred and treated?
- *Effectiveness*. Which treatment procedure produces a consistent increase in functional performance? How many therapy sessions are required to gain a satisfactory outcome?
- *Efficiency*. Which assessment best defines key problem areas quickly? Can some information be given to the patient in a written form prior to contact to reduce the amount of time given over to explanations?
- *Value*. Do the treatment gains result in reduced costs (e.g. reduced hospital stay), greater quality of life, or higher patient satisfaction?

Once the audit question has been formulated measures need to be specified which can act as the baseline for investigation. For example, outcome measures using standardised assessments giving pre- and post-treatment scores might be used. Alternatively the process of service delivery might be evaluated against set service *standards* or *protocols*.

For further information on clinical audit, see De Clive-Lowe (1996) or Spreadbury and Cook (1996).

Evaluating ourselves

Sometimes we are so busy assessing and caring for patients that we forget to assess and care for ourselves. Reflecting on our own performance, attitudes and actions is an anxiety-provoking business but it is crucial to our ability to work effectively in the long term. 'The most important prerequisite to being an effective helper is self-knowledge' (Hopkins and Tiffany, 1983, 94). In essence, we monitor ourselves to check standards of our past actions, gain support if needed for present activity and as a learning process for the future. The kinds of questions we regularly should ask ourselves include: Was my assessment of the patient fairly objective, with judgements backed by evidence? Did I have a clear overall view of treatment and proceed accordingly? Are my attitudes to my patient appropriate, or are negative feelings (e.g. pessimism, even hostility) getting in the way? Have I carried out the necessary team liaison to maintain relationships? What are my special strengths that I offer as a therapist?

We can evaluate ourselves in two main ways: through self-appraisal/reflection and through supervision/peer review.

Self-appraisal and reflection

Reflection can be described as 'emotion and action recollected in tranquillity' (Hagedorn, 1995, p. 191). Reflecting on our practice involves thinking about both how we feel and what we have done. Specifically we try to probe our behaviour, values and biases to see how these may have affected our treatment and relationships. All too often we ignore our subjective emotions yet they may well play a significant role in the therapy process.

Arguably our emotions can act as a useful barometer in our dealings with patients/clients. For example when we use a psychodynamic approach a key source of information involves analysing patients'/clients' transferences and our own counter-transferences. It may be equally valuable to examine our own reactions when working alongside co-therapists. Consider the Theory into Practice box below where a female group therapist reflects on her relationship with a male co-leader who is a doctor.

THEORY INTO PRACTICE

Reflecting on group dynamics and the co-leader relationship

I went into the group with some feelings of competition as my co-leader was a doctor. I was also ambivalent – grateful he wanted to work with me yet annoyed that he seemed to want to be a group leader as a research exercise rather than caring about the members. In the first group session, I had been going gently, trying to build up trust with this group of vulnerable women. Near the end of the session, Michael (co-leader) suddenly came out with what I perceived as a critical, insensitive remark. A female group member had just talked of her frustration that men only responded to her sexually. Michael confronted her saying she had a responsibility for this as she had even been giving him those messages. At that point the women in the group (including myself) felt furious! That feeling continued into the next group where the women were quite aggressive to Michael and I colluded by letting it happen. I was partially pleased because they were saying things I wanted to say. After the group, however, I thought about it and realised I had been unfair towards Michael. We sat down and properly shared our respective feelings. In doing so, our relationship as co-leaders was strengthened – an important step for the group as a whole.

Supervision and peer review

It is only by attending to our need for support and for learning that we are able to sustain the emotional and physical demands inherent in our work. Supervision and peer review can meet these needs, plus they offer an opportunity to evaluate one's own performance.

Ideally a formal supervision session (preferably with a senior colleague) should occur on a regular basis – say once a week. In addition therapists may need extra supervision to look specifically at difficult treatment sessions. The process of peer review can also be helpful as part of a wider supervision structure. Regular team meetings offer opportunities for both support and learning (e.g. meeting to discuss a case presentation or evaluate a course of groupwork). For further reading on these professional development issues, see Finlay (1993).

8.2 RESEARCH

Engelhardt has asserted that 'The unexamined profession is not worth practising' (Yerxa, 1986, p. 209) and this is as much true of occupational therapy as of any other profession. As therapists our practice would simply not be professional if we did not reflect on and evaluate our work. Professionals need to keep in touch with research and new developments in their field. We do this through: sharing our thoughts and practice with colleagues; carrying out our own investigations into whether or not our practice is effective and we also read about other peoples' experience and research.

Researchers contribute to our profession by developing our knowledge and guiding our theory. This helps us to refine our skills and evaluate our practice. Research has a way of questioning and challenging current, accepted practice; this can make us feel uneasy, and yet it is also that which challenges us to improve our service. Therefore the importance of research, for examining and substantiating our practice and for retaining professional credibility, cannot be overstated. Whilst not every occupational therapist will wish to be a 'research producer', we should all have a nodding acquaintance with its methods as a 'consumer'. In this sense research is within the reach and capabilities of all occupational therapists, however inexperienced we may be.

This research section will begin by asking why we need research. Secondly, two different research traditions will be examined – positivism (related to quantitative research) and naturalism (related to qualitative research). Thirdly, evaluation issues of validity, reliability and trustworthiness of research will be explored. Finally, tips for how to do research, either as a research consumer or a research producer, will be offered.

Why do we need to do research?

Research can be defined as any systematic activity which involves gathering information to answer a question. This may mean formal, large scale research projects (e.g. the type of studies which are reported in journals) or be at a less formal level (e.g. when we ask clients to fill out a feedback form/questionnaire at the end of a training course to survey their opinions). Reviewing the literature is another research activity (Stewart, 1990, calls this 'armchair research'). For example, if we wanted to carry out a standardised assessment (such as the Rivermead) but were inexperienced in its use, one thing we could do is check out old journal articles to see if any research had been carried out which could give clues to when to use it, with whom and how.

There are three good reasons why, as professionals, we need to do research.

1. Would you go to a doctor who prescribed an 'untested' medication? Would you be content to undergo a treatment that had no research backing it? Of course not, and nor would our patients/clients. Thus our *practice needs to be based on*

research. When we implement a specific treatment technique, we want to have confidence that it is likely to be effective, and know that it is underpinned by a strong empirical base (i.e. based on evidence).

2. We do research (armchair or otherwise) to be *informed and up-to-date* with trends, theories and practices. I know a therapist who absolutely refuses to read any of the literature that has come out in the last 10 years about the model of human occupation. To me, she is acting unprofessionally and this may prejudice her patients' treatment. She is also losing out on learning about many new assessments and research that have been based on the model. I do not say she has to adopt the model, but I do believe that she should investigate it prior to rejecting it. What's your view?

3. We do research to *gain from the experience* of others. For instance, a journal article which describes a treatment another therapist finds effective might well offer us some ideas for our own practice. Alternatively, we might gain insights into what not to do.

Two research traditions

Researchers in the social science field experience a tension between using concepts modelled on natural science (the so-called 'scientific method') and the idea that the social world is distinctive and somehow needs to be studied differently. This tension is presented here as a choice between two conflicting paradigms – positivism and naturalism. Decisions about whether to adopt a quantitative or qualitative approach to research emerges out of these two paradigms.

Positivism assumes reality consists of objectively definable facts. It privileges *quantitative* approaches to research and promotes the scientific method as espoused by natural science. Positivists seek to empirically test hypotheses through objective measurement. Positivist researchers aim to explain causal relationships and discover laws that can be generalised to wider populations and repeated to prove validity.

Naturalism (sometimes called the interpretive approach) believes in 'multiple realities' saying we each view the world differently. This means that objective measurement is virtually impossible and makes the discovery of fixed universal laws improbable. Naturalism leans towards *qualitative* approaches and favours research in natural settings (not laboratories). This tradition emphasises that human behaviour is dependent on social meanings (peoples' beliefs/feelings) which prompts individuals to act in unpredictable ways. Naturalist researchers aim to understand individuals within their own specific cultures. They prize subjectivity and richness of data instead of objectivity and measurement.

Quantitative versus qualitative approaches

Table 8.1 illustrates how the different approaches argue with each other in terms of their view of the social world, research methods, role of concepts/theory, data analysis and findings.

Table 8.1. Quantitative versus qualitative methods (adapted from Kielhofner, 1982, p. 69)

	Quantitative	*Qualitative*
View of the social world	A mechanistic stable order in which causal factors effect predictable outcomes; universal laws can be applied.	A dynamic, negotiated, situated order created by participants' meanings and actions.
Research method	Experiments observing behavioural responses; descriptive statistics; standardised tests; surveys and questionnaires.	Observations; participant observation; interviews; introspection and reflection; and analysis of documents.
Role of concepts/theory	Concepts operationalised into observable behaviours; deductive method where hypothesis testing leads to verification.	Sensitising concepts which capture individuals' meanings; inductive method where hypothesis and theory emerge last.
Data analysis	Experiments and surveys allow variables to be manipulated and relationships observed, then statistically analysed for probability.	Description and exploration of categories, themes and cultures with the aim of understanding.
Findings	Reliable and generalisable.	Rich with ecological validity.

Complementary or competing perspectives?

You can see from the above evaluation that quantitative and qualitative approaches have different strengths and weaknesses, so in a way they complement each other. Sometimes researchers will choose to mix quantitative and qualitative methods to offer different perspectives. For example, a researcher who surveys the views of 100 occupational therapists by way of questionnaire may supplement the data with some in-depth interviews to enrich understanding. Mixing methods in such a way may help the strengths and weaknesses of different approaches compensate for each other. However, be aware that the two approaches are also contradictory and it can be inappropriate (as well as unnecessary) to mix them.

Evaluating research

Validity, reliability and trustworthiness are fundamental requirements for sound research. Always check the extent to which the research measures what it sets out to measure (validity), that it measures it in a consistent way across time/raters (reliability), and that its methods and findings are well justified and open to scrutiny (trustworthiness).

Validity

Validity is probably best understood by applying it in practice. Here are two examples to think about:

Example 1
Say we set out to study the effectiveness of a relaxation exercise and used a biofeedback machine (a good measure of the extent of relaxation). This would be a potentially valid piece of research. Validity would be threatened however, if the subjects were sweating prior to being measured as it would not be clear if the result was due to exertion or stress level (Stewart, 1990).

Example 2
If we were studying whether or not patients' functioning improves after a specific treatment, we could observe/measure improvement by comparing pre- and post-treatment results using a standardised assessment. To ensure the assessment we are using offers a valid measure of the aspect we are assessing (for instance cognitive functioning), we might compare our test results with results gained from other cognitive function tests. Assuming the pattern of results is similar we can say our test has 'concurrent' validity.

Reliability

A reliable method is one which will produce same results if repeated (test–re-test reliability) or if applied by other researchers (inter-rater reliability). Reliability is often indicated by a correlation measure which varies from –1 to +1. For instance a correlation of +0.9 is extremely high and means there is a 90% chance the same scores will be obtained if the test is repeated. Think about a 'ruler' which is very reliable as different people measuring a length at different times, will (more or less) get the same result.

To illustrate this concept, consider some research on assessing patients before and after their treatment. If the researcher used a standardised assessment, we could be reasonably sure variations in data were due to changes in the patients' ability. If an unreliable tool had been used, any improvements could have occurred by chance or through researcher error/bias.

Trustworthiness

Positivist concepts of reliability and validity are inappropriate for evaluating qualitative research so the criteria of trustworthiness is usually employed. Reliability is irrelevant to qualitative research, by definition, since it does not seek to repeat research or obtain consistent accounts. An informant's responses are elicited within a specific and interpersonal context, and can never be replicated. Similarly, the goals of validity or generalisability are largely unachievable as single case studies cannot be representative of the whole population. Instead, qualitative researchers argue that they try to give enough detailed descriptions about the study to enable other researchers to use it as a basis of comparison.

Trustworthiness is argued, rather than proved, by systematically justifying claims. This is most commonly achieved using four methods:

Documented evidence
Documented evidence includes examples of behaviour and actual quotes (from informants or documents/records). The process of building comprehensive documents is important as it opens up the research to external audit. Thus a qualitative researcher will try to offer an account of their reasoning: Here is what my informant said. This is how I'm interpreting it and why. Is the story coherent and credible? What evidence can I supply to back up my interpretations so that others can confirm the plausibility of the study?

Reflexivity
Reflexivity can be defined as 'disciplined self-reflection' (Wilkinson, 1988, p. 493). Here the researcher reflects both on his/her own behaviour and about the research, trying to be aware of how his/her values/biases/interests influenced the research. The researcher's thinking needs to be fully acknowledged and revealed because they are part of the world they are studying.

Informant validation
Some qualitative researchers argue that one crucial test of validity is gaining the participants' endorsement of the researcher's interpretations. The value of informant validation is that it strengthens the claim that findings are not simply a product of author bias. At a philosophical level it is also consistent with the humanistic values underlying naturalism. There are considerable problems with this practice, however. For one thing informants may not feel able to disagree with the researcher. Even if they do, they may not have insight into their own behaviour or it may be in their interests to misrepresent themselves. We cannot say something is true simply because that is what the informant says.

Triangulation
Triangulation is the use of different vantage points to exploit combinations of informants, investigators or methods. The validity of a study's conclusions can be strengthened when several informants or researchers offer similar accounts or interpretations. Similarly, researchers who mix methods can have more confidence that their data is more than simply the product of their method. The argument against triangulation is that getting such extra data may be unnecessary and confusing. 'More' is not necessarily 'better'. For example, an analysis can become

very messy if several researchers employ their own interpretations and preferred models of understanding.

On being a research consumer – critiquing research

The first step on the ladder of 'doing research' is being an interested consumer. Regularly reading (and critically analysing) various research papers is an excellent way of both tuning into current issues and grappling with the methods, jargon and concepts of research. A good place to start is the *British Journal of Occupational Therapy*, which regularly publishes research papers. Other occupational therapy journals of note include the American, Canadian and Australian occupational therapy journals, the *Occupational Therapy Journal of Research*, and the *Journal of Occupational Science*. The new *Mental Health OT* magazine contains a number of short, topical articles will also be of interest to psycho-social therapists. In addition, journals/periodicals from nursing, psychiatry, rehabilitation and the social sciences offer much that is potentially exciting and relevant. The notion of literature searches or coping with library technology can seem a daunting prospect for the uninitiated. However, it gets easier as you work at it and, once mastered, the pursuit of questions and answers can be fun.

Once you embark on reading research, it can be quite daunting to try to make sense of an article let alone evaluate it critically. It takes skill, knowledge and a positive, questioning attitude to evaluate research and it is not a simple technique we pick up over night. One of the first lessons is to note both strengths and weaknesses of an article (Finlay, 1997). Not all research is valid or trustworthy – sometimes it can be misleading or biased. If you were reading about research on a new drug, would not you be slightly cautious about the findings on discovering the research was produced by the manufacturers? In much the same way if you read in a professional journal that a new theory/assessment is brilliant, would you believe it without question?

Most research is ethical and authors work hard to ensure their findings and presentations are objective and trustworthy. However, even this research needs to be critically examined. If you read of some research about an occupational therapy technique would you just import its ideas into your practice? I suspect not – instead you would think about the research and how it might apply in your particular situation. You would consider what insights it offered, what was useful to you about the technique and when/how you might implement it.

THEORY INTO PRACTICE

Questions to ask when critiquing research

Research context
What is the research all about?
Are the research aims and hypotheses/questions clearly laid out?

To what extent is the link to theory and previous research explained?
How interesting and relevant is the research?
What are the implications and value of the research?
Are there ethical implications and have these been handled appropriately?

Data collection

(a) Subjects and setting
　　Who are the research subjects and setting?
　　How were these selected?
　　To what extent will the findings generalise to wider populations/situations?

(b) Methods and procedures
　　Are the details spelt out sufficiently to allow the study to be replicated?
　　How appropriate are the methods and procedures adopted?
　　What steps were taken to ensure validity/reliability or trustworthiness of the results?

Data analysis

How clearly are the results presented and discussed?
If any statistics are used are they appropriate to the research design?
Is the link between the data and results well argued?
How comprehensive is the discussion?
Does the discussion relate sufficiently to both the research questions and literature review?
Are the author's conclusions logical and valid?
Have other competing hypotheses and explanations been recognised?
Does the author offer critical evaluation of his/her own methodology?
Has anything significant been left out?

Write up

Is it clearly and appropriately structured?
Is the writing style accessible?
Is the structure and use of language appropriate to the type of research? (Finlay, 1997).

On being a research producer

Occupational therapy research in the UK is still in its early stages but it is an area that is fast expanding as more of us get involved. Increasingly, occupational therapists are gaining research experience either in pursuit of research degrees or because of the changes that have occurred in our basic training, where research is now automatically included. This is set within the backdrop of pressure to produce evidence for, and to evaluate our service in response to, quality assurance programmes.

So what research can we usefully carry out? For a start, it is particularly important for us to 'prove' the benefit and effectiveness of our treatment activities. A wide range of different types of research is possible. Consider the following examples for some ideas – all of which are likely to be of interest and of use to our profession.

- *Experiment.* Compare three matched groups of patients. Group 1 receives treatment 'A' (e.g. relaxation group). Group 2 receives treatment 'B' (e.g. education/information about anxiety management). Group 3 is the control group and does not receive any particular treatment.
- *Survey.* Do a descriptive study surveying clients' attitudes to their treatment activities using a standard questionnaire.
- *Interview.* Carry out in-depth interviews of clients in the community about their mental health and treatment experiences.
- *Participant observation.* Join a 'self-help' group and through using observation and personal reflection analyse the experience and benefits of being in the group.

How do we carry out research? The process is a complex one requiring much organisation and knowledge of correct method. Thus it is always best, for the first time at least, to be well supervised or work with an experienced colleague/team. For a highly readable account of how to do research, I recommend Drummond (1996).

THEORY INTO PRACTICE

Summary of 'how to do research'

1. *Background thinking/organisation.* Read round the subject; refine ideas; decide on a research question and design; carry out necessary liaison.
2. *Prepare research method.* Consider methods, resources, reliability, validity, trustworthiness; prepare measurement tools.
3. *Collect data.* Run pilot and make adjustments; collect real data ensuring accuracy and ethical aspects (confidentiality, not harming patients, rights to privacy).
4. *Analyse results.* Explain clearly by thematic analysis or by using relevant tables, graphs, statistical analysis, etc.; recognise implications.
5. *Present results.* Write up in the following format: title; abstract; introduction and review of literature; procedures/methods; results and discussion or thematic analysis; conclusion; and references.

At the end of the day you should be able to answer the following questions:

Questions	*Sections in your report*
Why did I start?	Introduction and objectives
What did I do?	Methodology
What answer did I get?	Results and analysis
What does it mean?	Discussion and conclusions

One last point concerning being a research producer that should be stressed is the importance of publishing research. A researcher may feel he or she is taking a risk of having the work open to scrutiny by others – but even if the feedback is critical, will this not be useful for future projects? Furthermore, it is only through publishing our material that we can share our knowledge and labours, thus gaining from each other. For those interested, copies of Master's and Doctoral level theses written by occupational therapists are available from: DISC, the College of Occupational Therapists, 6–8 Marshalsea Road, London SE1 1HL.

CONCLUSION

This chapter has explored a range of tools for evaluating our practice – from tools to evaluate patients' progress, treatment, service delivery and our own performance, through to long-term research. I have stressed the need to undertake evaluation systematically (e.g. using standard measures and engage in careful clinical audit and valid research). However, we must not lose sight of the value of subjective measures such as self-report and reflection. It is only by combining these methods can we hope to come close to evaluating the full complexity and richness of occupational therapy practice.

For the future we can anticipate exciting initiatives for evaluating and researching practice. Yerxa has written about the 'evolution of professional knowledge which proceeds from the intuitive practice of an untested art to the logically rigorous practice of a science.' (Hopkins and Smith, 1983, p. 872). Perhaps we should strive to achieve a balance between the two. Certainly we need to develop more reliable instruments and ways of testing our practice. At the same time we need to retain our humanistic values and holistic concerns. We need to avoid reducing our patients to experimental subjects and viewing them in terms of inappropriately narrow outcome measurements. The challenge lies in finding methods to suit our practice, as well as adapting our practice in the light of the findings from our evaluations.

Discussion questions

1. What measures are available to evaluate a patient's/client's progress?
2. Should occupational therapists always use objective outcome measures?
3. Describe the range of tools available for evaluating treatment?
4. Why is it important that occupational therapists carry out research?
5. Critically evaluate a newly published research article of interest.
6. Analyse the different commitments and methodologies of the two research traditions of positivism and naturalism.

Professional themes and issues

In recent years the wider health care service has been significantly reshaped. Many forces have contributed to these developments including: new ideologies about the role of the health service; the philosophy of care in the community; the rise of new technologies; shifting demography and changes in professional education.

These changes have radically affected occupational therapy. We have adapted in ways that have sometimes been difficult and sometimes put us at the forefront of innovation. Many of these trends have been touched on in earlier chapters. This chapter focuses on these and aims to stimulate discussion. It is an opportunity to articulate both the problems and pressures we face and to indicate the excitements and opportunities they open up for us. Our profession is embroiled in a process of continuous, fast change. Awareness of these issues is essential if we are to meet future developments positively and constructively.

This chapter reflects on how developments in health care have impacted on our profession. In order to give some logic to our exploration of current and future trends, I have selected four themes for discussion. The first three relate to the continuing drive towards practice that is systematic, client-centred and community-orientated. The fourth stresses the need to continue to promote occupational therapy in the wider world. I end with some thoughts about our future role and functions.

HEALTHCARE CONTEXT AND THE OCCUPATIONAL THERAPIST'S ROLE

The last decade has witnessed dramatic changes in the UK health care context. We have experienced major structural and economic reorganisation with the development of Trust status, management systems, GP fund-holding and the separation of purchaser–provider–consumer concerns in health planning. Along with the ideology of the (mixed) market have come calls for efficiency, cost effectiveness and value for money in healthcare. Hospital closures and the development of private and community based medicine have catapulted both the local authority and the voluntary sector further into the health care arena.

Some claim the National Health Service is in financial crisis and on the point of collapse, others point to the extra public spending the health service has soaked up in recent years. New technologies, expensive treatments and the rise in patient demand have continued to put pressure on the health service. Further pressure comes from shifting demographics, i.e. the acute and growing problem of our rapidly ageing population. Health service planners and providers are being forced into tough decisions about priority setting. The division of care between health and social services, where each seeks to limit costs, has caused some patients/clients to fall into the middle ground between the two services. This has resulted in calls for greater attention to be paid to the total 'spectrum of care'.

On the positive side, our health service has become more efficient and stream-lined. The increasing emphasis on clinical audit and greater accountability has undoubtedly raised our standards as we seek to demonstrate professional quality and effectiveness. Also, there have been forward strides in both research and innovation. Further, most agree that the idea (if not the practice) of community care is essentially a humane and healthy way forward.

All of these changes have had (and will continue to have) considerable impact on our professional practice. First, the new imperatives of clinical effectiveness and cost efficiency have created a number of pressures for us (even to the point of being forced into competing for jobs). We are being asked to demonstrate our value. Could some of our work be carried out by (cheaper) support staff? Could other professional groups (e.g. nurses) do what we do plus other things like give out medication? Currently there is still a shortage of occupational therapists but if we want to survive as a profession in the long run we must be able to prove our effectiveness and promote our role. The question remains do we have a unique occupational therapy contribution to make or could a generic therapist offer a more effective service?

Secondly, health care changes have resulted in much internal reorganisation. Posts have been restructured (even down-graded) and there has been a breakdown of traditional professional hierarchies. Occupational therapists are no longer always managed by their own profession. At one level this has meant the loss of vital supervision and support (to say nothing of a traditional promotional structure). At another level it has brought benefits as we have been forced to collaborate with, and so learn from, others. Different opportunities have opened up alongside new promotion structures (e.g. becoming involved with research or general management).

Thirdly, our role within the treatment team continues to evolve, particularly as we forge new community teams and practices. Increasingly, we find ourselves operating as a single, possibly isolated, professional in the team. Lacking profession-specific support, it is not surprising some therapists have lost a sense of our particular occupational therapy contribution and instead favour more generic practices such as counselling. Thus, we have seen the growth of occupational therapists taking on positions such as 'care managers', 'key workers' and 'mental health or clinical practitioners'. A positive spin off from this has been closer teamwork and thus more effective treatment. With these new challenges have come learning opportunities as we have shared skills and collaborated in research. Furthermore, being separated from rigid role definitions allows us the flexibility to forge new practices with a view to offering the ideal of a spectrum of care.

TOWARDS A MORE SYSTEMATIC PRACTICE?

In this era of greater accountability we are constantly being asked to justify our work and assure its quality. In practice this means that we need to be specific about our aims and outcome measures, carry out treatments in a coherent manner and evaluate our service in a comprehensive way. It also requires us to emphasise the value of the contributions our profession makes to health care both now and in the future. What is more we must learn to communicate this as clearly and vigorously as possible, particularly when we come to present reports and argue for more resources. These are imperatives and point to the need for us to be more systematic in our work and more scientific in our methodology.

Said quickly, this all sounds easy. Yet buried beneath are complexities which pose many problems. Let us start with the notion of quality assurance – now a common concept which draws on models of efficiency, productivity and higher standards of service derived from industry. Certainly there are some parallels between industry and occupational therapy. Both need efficient organisation and require clear objectives and outcome measures against which to evaluate their work. Yet there are also important differences between commercial product production and caring. These must not be ignored. Communal systems for service delivery and resource management may benefit us whilst techniques of door to door selling will not. We must learn to draw selectively and qualitatively on systems which will enhance our goals.

A major hurdle we face, in attempting to assure quality, is to identify precisely what we are trying to do. There are two reasons why this is so difficult. First, our practice is diverse, given our varying theoretical bases, roles, concerns and work contexts. Secondly, it is not an easy task to quantify our therapeutic input and measure output given that we deal with many largely unquantifiable processes and have yet to discover some basic tools for meaningful measurement of effectiveness. How can we define our approach to, and relationship with, individual patients/clients? How can we adequately measure the social and affective aspects of the therapy process? Can we even identify what particular aspect of our use of activity is therapeutic? When a person gains from occupational therapy often the gain is not measurable, such as when the person says 'I feel I'm coping better'.

These are some of the difficulties we face, particularly in mental health, when attempting to specify our service.

However, to argue that our work cannot easily be defined, monitored or measured does not mean that we should not try to make an effort in this direction where it is appropriate to do so. There are for example some obvious and concrete tasks, that we can undertake for ourselves as a profession, which will ultimately lead to an improvement in our service to our patients/clients. We can:

- Be clear and systematic when we are identifying patients'/clients' problems and the aims/objectives and methods of their treatment.
- Use and develop standardised assessments enabling us to more accurately identify individuals' functioning and measure progress.
- Research and develop different models and tools to measure process and outcomes.
- Record/report information more accurately and engage in clinical audit exercises – taking the risk of having our work open to scrutiny by others.
- Adopt standards and protocols (whilst maintaining a client-centred approach) which can be evaluated through audit.
- Encourage the development of research and evidence based practice to both substantiate our present and direct our future practices in a more theoretically sophisticated and scientifically justifiable way.
- Undertake post-professional education, for instance up-dating knowledge by attending conferences or doing research towards a higher degree.
- Reflect on the role and practice of occupational therapy and take the opportunities to debate the state of our profession and the shape of its future development. We should move away from pondering the question 'what is occupational therapy?' and start asking 'what should or will occupational therapy be? What do we want to make it?'

TOWARDS A MORE PERSON-CENTRED PRACTICE?

If we need to move towards becoming more systematic and rigorous in our approach to occupational therapy, we need simultaneously to focus on the 'person' behind the patient – paying increasing attention to his or her individuality, rights and needs.

This can be seen at several levels. First, in keeping with our holistic philosophy we need to move away (and are doing so) from reductionist views of medical and behavioural models which depersonalise with labels and diagnoses. Instead we should pay more attention to the individual's situation and recognise that illness is only one small aspect of the whole person. When we do use a diagnosis we need to try to preserve the human element in our definitions and our verbal usages. Consider the simple but profound difference between saying 'the person with a diagnosis of schizophrenia', as against 'that schizophrenic'. Behind this difference in semantics lies some very important differences in attitudes towards concepts of health and illness, and the extent to which the physical, emotional and social impact of our treatments are taken into account.

A further key part of this recognition of the individual is the need to plan an individualised treatment based on an assessment of a person's specific needs, interests and values. The days when we received blanket referrals for all patients to attend the department, for whatever activity currently in progress, have long gone. Whilst limited resources may hamper the extent to which individual treatment planning is possible for all patients/clients, attempts to move in this direction must be made. Many departments, for example, now run a range of activities into which patients/clients are carefully and selectively referred. Increasingly we are trying to 'fit our service to the patient', rather than 'patients to our service'.

Another facet of this recognition of the specificity of an individual's situation is also the need to acknowledge the differences between people's social and cultural background. Many occupational therapists now work in multi-cultural areas where it is vital that they are aware of the particular needs of different ethnic groups (e.g. religious customs, values and taboos). Equally, we need to consider the impact of class, gender, race and age on a person's life chances, given the widespread patterns of disadvantage and even discrimination that exist with regard to them. We need to take all this into account if we are going to plan treatments that are both relevant and realistic in today's climate.

Lastly, the patient/client needs to be seen as the key member of the treatment team. Fundamental to this notion is the need to plan treatment *with* our patients/clients, rather than regard them as the passive recipients of our service. This concept can be taken further to stress the importance of the idea of offering people, i.e. the consumers, choices. This is a particularly acute issue when an individual is being forced against his or her will to come to occupational therapy, or is coerced into activity. This is clearly undesirable, and alerts us to the need to ask ourselves what the individual sees as 'in his or her interest'. If our patients/clients are unable to specify their choice and interest, we need to take extra care to act in the role of their advocate (perhaps in conjunction with their carers). Increasingly therapists are taking on this role, particularly in instances where their clients have unfair and unequal access to care, resources or opportunities.

TOWARDS COMMUNITY PRACTICE

Over the last decade government papers (e.g. the Griffiths Report *Community Care: Agenda for Action* and *Caring for People: Community Care in the Next Decade and Beyond*) and legislation (in the form of the National Health Service and Community Care Act, 1990) has promoted care in the community. As hospitals close, patients get discharged quicker and new community-orientated services open, the face of therapy services has changed. New community teams have been formed and hospital-based therapists have reorientated their focus towards providing a spectrum of care.

The current comunity focus offers exciting opportunities for the development of our profession given our central focus on people's lifestyles and daily living skills. We are not as constrained as other professions who are still required to provide hospital based acute care. I believe most occupational therapists would favour being involved in the full spectrum of care where we can follow-up clients in the community as well as see them through hospital admissions and out again. Community centred practice like this has taken off. Many hospital based therapists now carry an out-patient caseload, whilst community therapists stress liaison with hospital services.

The implications of such changes for our actual practice are enormous:

1. With the trend towards shorter admissions, hospital based occupational therapists have moved away from supplying treatment activities for the here and now and are increasingly focused on *managing discharge*. In order to act as a bridge from hospital to community, therapists are now following up patients after they are discharged (e.g. setting up out-patient groups).
2. The nature of our work has shifted from doing group activity treatment in hospital to offering more one-to-one interventions in the client's home.
3. Increasingly, we are less involved in doing activities directly with clients. Instead we aim to enable them to be active (e.g. teaching them to use local leisure facilities).
4. Occupational therapists working under different guises such as 'care manager' or 'clinical practitioner' can be found in many different community settings based in community teams, day units and residential homes.
5. We are becoming increasingly involved in primary care and supporting clients in the community in an effort to prevent hospital admission. To this end we are becoming attached to primary care teams including GP services.

I believe these developments are here to stay, and that we should embrace them positively and pro-actively. We also need to shift our understanding of our role in community rehabilitation. First, as the burden of care for people increasingly falls on families and the local community, occupational therapists need to respond to this. We have a two-pronged role: (a) to support the carers and (b) to act as the client's advocate, particularly in the face of hostile community reactions. Secondly, with hospital based rehabilitation programmes diminishing, the demand for rehabilitation in the community rises. Currently there are large gaps in treatment provision, particularly for the increasing numbers of people with long-term disabilities. Occupational therapists are well placed to respond to this demand and need to fight for more community based day units which offer vital social support and productive 'work' or activity opportunities. We should aim to become 'disability or lifestyle managers' (Richards, 1996).

TOWARDS PROMOTING OCCUPATIONAL THERAPY

Occupational therapists must fight for recognition and resources. This is not new. In the past, we have fought many battles, yet today, particularly in the context of increasing competition for limited health resources and the trend towards multi-disciplinary role-blurring, there are as many threats to our growth as ever. Our motive for promoting occupational therapy cannot simply be anchored in professional self-interest or our corporate history. Ultimately it is dependent upon us being proud of what we do, and wanting to share it with others.

How often do we complain about not being taken seriously as professionals? How often do we feel discouraged because occupational therapy seems undervalued and no-one appears interested in what we say in ward rounds? Whilst the way our profession is perceived varies enormously from place to place, many of us are still in the business of challenging the false or even negative images of occupational therapy which others sometimes have. At the same time it has to be recognised that some, at least, of these negative images may be the result of the way we have presented ourselves in the past. Herein lies the need for us to promote occupational therapy – and promote it in several directions, not only towards the general public, but also, in the direction of patients/clients and the treatment team.

The general public has a limited and confused view of what we do. Likewise often our patients/clients come to us feeling unsure about what we offer, or unmotivated because of some inadequate image that, for instance, 'occupational therapy is just about keeping people occupied'. It is crucial that we explain occupational therapy to our patients/clients to enable them to feel reassured and clear about what they can gain from our treatments. Succinct and relevant explanations should always be offered in the early stages of treatment. A simple statement on the following lines might help to ease their doubts and will help to get them involved in their own treatment from the beginning: 'I'm concerned with how you cope with your everyday activities – at work, at home or in terms of caring for yourself and having a satisfying social life ...'; alternatively, 'Occupational therapy is a treatment which aims to help people cope with different problems they may be having. We do lots of different things. Why not come down to the department with me and have a look around and talk to some of the patients there?'. The main point is to try to make the explanation most relevant to the individuals concerned. They do not need to know about occupational therapy so much as knowing how it could apply to them.

The rest of the treatment team also needs to know about, and recognise the value of, occupational therapy. At one level they are important ambassadors for us; for instance, when explaining our role to an uncertain patient. At another level the team needs to be clear about our functions (and we about their functions) to enable smooth liaison and co-operative effort. This task of educating colleagues needs to be done continuously at both formal (e.g. when presenting a report at a case conference) and informal (e.g. when chatting casually on the ward with nurses) levels. It is important to remember also the outward impression we may give when we invite visitors/team members/students around the department – additional explanations, for example of the aims of treatment activity taking place, are essential.

At a more instrumental or political level our image and perceived role within a unit or hospital (and within the management hierarchy) matters if we are to maintain, or attract more of, the resources which are necessary to enable us to do our job effectively. Here, again, we need to communicate with others both widely and well. Writing reports, making presentations, holding open days, producing leaflets, etc., all involve some degree of presenting and promoting occupational therapy to a wider audience. Beyond marketing ourselves we must be clear about the value/benefit of what we offer and demonstrate that our practice is backed by sound evidence and research. Most of all, we promote our profession by doing a good job.

REFLECTING ON THE FUTURE

As we move into the new millennium, how is our professional practice likely to develop? I believe all of the themes discussed above (i.e. the emphasis on systematic, person-centred community practice) will continue to be relevant. In terms of what we specifically *do*, I would like to suggest four main shifts in our emphasis.

First, our *role* is likely to continue to develop away from being a therapist towards acting as a consultant. The significant point here is that we are likely to be less involved in actually carrying out treatment. Instead we will co-ordinate treatment; supervise and manage support staff as they do the 'hands on'; and enable clients themselves to be active. Rather than teaching a client pottery, we will encourage them to go to a class in the community. We will have a key role to play in mobilising community support systems (e.g. using voluntary agencies and working with carers).

Secondly, our focus on clients' *leisure and work* will continue to evolve. Although the types of leisure pursuits will change (see below related to technology), our aim to develop clients' leisure pursuits will clearly continue.. The role of 'paid work' will be less important than productivity in general (i.e. attendance at various activity centres and domestic or voluntary work). Where we are involved in work rehabilitation we will need to recognise the demands of different work patterns (e.g. part-time and casual employment).

Thirdly, the role and *use of technology* will continue to expand and this may well open up a serious gap between therapists with technical expertise and others who lack it. Already many units use computer games (to develop cognitive and task performance) and videos (for groupwork and family therapy). The use of computer technology will grow in significance and can be seen at different levels. In the first place we will be confronted with the fact that an increasing number of our patients/clients use computers in their daily lives (for both leisure and work). How can we ignore this? At another level, as we rehabilitate and resettle people in the community we need to address their basic skills which will include the ability to use basic computer technology (e.g. cash card machines, and programming videos, ansamachines and satellite TVs).

The growth of computer use in the form of the Internet/World Wide Web and E-mail is also likely to alter all of our lives. Clients may well draw on the Internet for social interaction and support. Therapists will use it increasingly to communicate with other team members and to network with colleagues around the world. Just to make this point, check out the Internet pages related to occupational therapy. Two particularly useful pages are currently listed as:

- 'OT Internet Links' page = http://www.iop.bpmf.ac.uk/home/sha/ot/otlinks.htm
- Association of Occupational Therapists in Mental Health Internet page = http:/www.iop.bpmf.ac.uk/home/trust/ot/aotmh.htm (Chacksfield, 1996).

Finally, the Commission chaired by Louis Blom-Cooper from the late 1980s produced its report: *Occupational Therapy: An Emerging Profession in Health Care* (Blom-Cooper, 1989). The report recognised we are still finding our professional role and identity. The Commission urged occupational therapists to prepare for new opportunities in the community acknowledging our role in maximising clients' daily living skills and independence as well as enabling meaningful quality of life. These continue to be our strengths upon which the profession can build. Do we believe in what we have to offer? Are we up for the challenge?

*   *   *   *   *   *   *   *   *   *   *   *

In this and the preceding chapters we have tried to unravel some of the complexities of our occupational therapy process and give examples of our work in practice. We have stressed themes such as the need to be both systematic and scientific while also remaining person-centred and sensitive to the needs of our patients within the treatment process. We have explored a number of the dilemmas arising from our multi-faceted role and our wide theoretical base. The intention has been to be informative and to spark off some interest and debate. Throughout all of these discussions, what has been offered is only one way of carrying out psychosocial occupational therapy (the way that makes sense to me given my experiences). It does not claim to be the only way. You may well find other, hopefully better, ways. We are not dealing with a clear-cut subject which has any easy or stereotyped answers. Instead, we may take many perspectives and focus in on problems and treatments at different levels.

Yes, occupational therapy in mental health can be utterly confusing, filled with ambiguities, contradictions, frustrations and stresses. We have relatively few answers and are often baffled by the complexities of the people and problems with which we have to deal. On the other hand, occupational therapy in mental health can be endlessly interesting, thought-provoking, and even fun. We can experience the sense of satisfaction and professional fulfilment when a person's treatment actually works out as we had hoped, or take pleasure in a certain activity or relationship that feels just 'right'. The experience of sharing in someone's growth and development, of enabling someone (in however small a way) to cope better, somehow makes it all worthwhile. Occupational therapy offers a continuous challenge, opportunities and rich rewards.

Appendix

INTEREST CHECKLIST (MODIFIED) INDICATING ONLY ITEMS TO WHICH JACK RESPONDED POSITIVELY (SEE CASE ILLUSTRATION 2.1: JACK)

Activity	Past interest level	Current participation	Future participation
Playing cards	some	no	maybe
Walking	some	no	yes
Football	high	watches on TV	yes
Swimming	was interested to learn	no	would like to learn
Reading	likes reading newspaper	yes	yes
Television	high	favourite activity	yes
Pottery	was interested to learn	no	would like to learn
Other – going to pubs	some	no	yes probably

II | **Appendix**

RECORD OF ACTIVITY (SEE CASE ILLUSTRATION 2.1: JACK)

Initial assessment – Jack's typical Saturday

10:00 am	Lie in bed; eventually get up; have cereal for breakfast; wash up.
10:30–12:30	Sit in chair.
12:30	Eat dinner which wife cooks; help wash up perhaps with a daughter.
1:30–5:00	Nap in chair and watch TV.
5:00–9:00	Tea; watch TV; go to bed.

Towards end of treatment – Jack's typical Saturday

9:00 am	Lie in bed; eventually get up; have cereal for breakfast; wash up.
10:00	Go for walk and buy a newspaper.
11:00	Prepare dinner or help wife.
12:00	Dinner and help wash up.
1:00–5:00	Watch sports or go on outing with family (e.g. swimming).
5:00–11:00	Tea; watch TV; go to bed.

Appendix

III

VALUES CHECKLIST (DONE VERBALLY AND MODIFIED TO BE APPROPRIATE FOR JACK'S LEVEL OF UNDERSTANDING)

Five activities I really enjoy doing	Why is it a good activity?
Pottery	I can make things that are good and give them to my family. They think I'm clever.
Swimming	It's nice to do. I've always wanted to learn since I was a child.
Coming to occupational therapy	I like it here. Mike (staff member) is my friend and is very good. I like to work.
Cooking	I like to eat the things. They taste nice. My family like what I cook too.
Outings with family	I don't know.

Appendix

**THE OCCUPATIONAL PERFORMANCE HISTORY INTERVIEW
RATING AND LIFE HISTORY NARRATIVE FORM**

Name: EDNA   Date:

Interviewer:

DEMARCATION OF PAST/PRESENT

——Six-month default/anchoring point

OR

——Specific event circumstance. How far in past   /   11

                                                     year(s)   months

Nature of event/circumstance   Death of spouse

            (☐ = Score before spouse's stroke 15 years ago)

OCCUPATIONAL PERFORMANCE HISTORY RATING SCALE

Circle the number that best characterizes the individual's adaptive status or environmental influences for each key item in both past and present.

		PAST	PRESENT
ADAPTIVE STATUS OF THE INDIVIDUAL	*1. Organisation of Daily Living Routines*		
	Maintaining organised functional daily routines	[5] (4) 3 2 1	5 4 3 (2) 1
	Balancing work, play and daily living tasks	[5] 4 (3) 2 1	5 4 3 2 (1)
	2. Life Roles		
	Maintaining involvement in life roles	[5] 4 (3) 2 1	5 4 3 2 (1)
	Fulfilment of expectations of life roles	[5] (4) 3 2 1	5 4 3 2 (1)
	3. Interests, Values and Goals		
	Identifying interests, values and goals	[5] (4) 3 2 1	5 (4) 3 2 1
	Enacting interests, values and goals	5 [4] 3 (2) 1	5 4 3 2 (1)
	4. Perception of Ability and Responsibility		
	Recognising abilities and limitations	[5] 4 (3) 2 1	5 4 (3) 2 1
	Taking on responsibility	[5] 4 3 2 1	5 4 (3) 2 1
ENVIRONMENT	*5. Environment Influences*		
	Influences of the human environment	[5] 4 (3) 2 1	5 (4) 3 2 1
	Influences of the nonhuman environment	[5] 4 3 2 1	5 (4) 3 2 1

After Keilhofner *et al.* (1989).

V	**Appendix**

INTERACTION OF OCCUPATIONAL BEHAVIOUR AND COMPONENTS OF SKILLS

	ADL: hygiene, dressing, eating, health maintenance, community mobility	Productive Activities: work, voluntary work, domestic management, education, caring for others	Leisure Activities: play, socialisation, hobby/interests, creative expresession
	OCCUPATIONAL BEHAVIOUR		
Sensory Motor Aspects sensory motor neuromuscular			
Cognitive Aspects orientation attention activity engagement memory sequencing problem solving learning			
Psychological Aspects emotional social self-management			

COMPONENTS OF SKILLS

This grid is a modified and summarised version of the one which appears in *American Occupational Therapy Association* (1994). The two axes in that version are entitled 'performance areas' and 'performance components'. I recommend returning to this original source to appreciate the full grid with all its extra details.

The grid can be used as an analytical devise in which therapists conceptualise occupational behaviour as being constituted by task and interpersonal skill components. Equally on identifying skill deficits in an individual, the therapist could work across the grid to understand which parts of the person's occupational behaviour are affected. For one example of how to apply this grid, see Hansen and Atchinson (1993).

References

Ager, A. (1990) *Life Experiences Checklist*. NFER-Nelson, Windsor, Berkshire.

Alexander, B. K. (1990) The empirical and theoretical bases for an adaptive model of addiction. *The Journal of Drug Issues*, 20, 37–65.

Allen, C. K. (1985) *Occupational Therapy for Psychiatric Diseases: Measurement and Management of Cognitive Disabilities*. Little, Brown and Co., Boston, MA.

American Occupational Therapy Association (1994) Uniform terminology for occupational therapists, 3rd edn. *American Journal of Occupational Therapy*, **48**, 1047–1054.

Axline, V. (1971) *Dibs: In Search of Self*. Penguin, Harmondsworth.

Axline, V. (1989) *Play Therapy*. Churchill Livingstone, Edinburgh.

Baron, K. B. (1994) Clinical interpretation of 'the Assessment of Motor and Process Skills of persons with psychiatric disorders'. *American Journal of Occupational Therapy*, **48**, 781–782.

Bion, W. R. (1961) *Experiences in Groups and other Papers*. Tavistock, London.

Blair, S. (1990) Occupational therapy and group psychotherapy. In J. Creek (ed.), *Occupational Therapy and Mental Health*, Churchill Livingstone, Edinburgh.

Blom-Cooper, L. (1989) *Occupational Therapy: An Emerging Profession in Health Care*. Duckworth, London.

Borg, B. and Bruce, M. A. (1991) *The Group System: The Therapeutic Activity Group in Occupational Therapy*. Slack, Thorofare, NJ.

Bowlby, J. (1971) *Attachment and Loss. Vol. 1: Attachment*. Pelican, Harmondsworth.

Bowlby, J. (1975) *Separation, Anxiety and Anger*. Pelican, Harmondsworth.

Bracegirdle, H. (1996) Developing physical fitness to promote mental health. In J. Creek (ed.), *Occupational Therapy and Mental Health*, 2nd edn. Churchill Livingstone, Edinburgh.

Brayman, S. J., Kirby, T. F., Misenheimer, A. M. and Short, M. J. (1976) Comprehensive occupational therapy evaluation scale. *American Journal of Occupational Therapy*, **30**, 94–100.

Briggs, A. K., Duncombe, L. W., Howe, M. C. and Schwartzberg, S. L. (1979) *Case Simulations in Psychosocial Occupational Therapy*. Davis, Philadelphia, PA.

Burton, J. (1989) The model of human occupation and occupational therapy practice with elderly patients, part 2: application. *British Journal of Occupational Therapy*, **52**, 219–221.

Canadian Association of Occupational Therapists (1991) *Occupational Therapy Guidelines for Client-Centred Practice*. Canadian Association of Occupational Therapists Publications, Toronto.

Chacksfield, J. (1996) Technology: making the Internet connection – the AOTMH page and Ots on the Internet. *Mental Health OT*, **1**, 23–25.

Chern, J., Kielhofner, G., Heras, C. and Magaheas, L. (1996) The Volitional Questionnaire: psychometric development and practical use. *American Journal of Occupational Therapy*, **50**, 516–525.

Christiansen, C. and Baum, C. (1991) *Occupational Therapy: Overcoming Performance Deficits*. Slack, Thorofare, NJ.

Clark, D. M. (1986) A cognitive approach to panic. *Behaviour Research and Therapy*, **24**, 461–470.

Clark, D. M., Salkovkskis, P. M., Hackmann, A., Middleton, H. L., Anastasiades, P. and Gelder, M. (1994) A comparison of cognitive therapy, applied relaxation and imipramine in the treatment of panic disorder. *British Journal of Psychiatry*, **164**, 759–769.

Coleman, P. (1986) *Ageing and Reminiscence Process*. John Wiley & Sons, Chichester.

Cox, W. M. and Klinger, E. (1988) A motivational model of alcohol abuse. *Journal of Abnormal Psychology*, **97**, 168–180.

Creek, J. (ed.) (1996) *Occupational Therapy and Mental Health*, 2nd edn. Churchill Livingstone, Edinburgh.

Creek, J. and Feaver, S. (1993) Models for practice in occupational therapy, part 1: defining terms. *British Journal of Occupational Therapy*, **56**, 4–6.

De Clive-Lowe, S. (1996) Outcome measurement, cost-effectiveness and clinical audit: the importance of standardised assessment to occupational therapists in meeting these new demands. *British Journal of Occupational Therapy*, **59**, 357–362.

De las Heras, C. G. (1995) *A User's Guide to the Volitional Questionnaire*. The University of Illinois at Chicago, Chicago, IL.

Drummond, A. (1996) *Research Methods for Therapists*. Chapman & Hall, London.

Eakin, P. (1989a) Assessments of activities of daily living: a critical review. *British Journal of Occupational Therapy*, **52**, 11–16.

Eakin, P. (1989b) Problems with assessments of activities of daily living. *British Journal of Occupational Therapy*, **52**, 50–54.

Egan, G. (1986) *The Skilled Helper*, 3rd edn. Brooks Cole, Monterey, CA.

Eisenbruch, M. (1993) 'Wind illness' or somatic depression? A case study in psychiatric anthropology. *British Journal of Psychiatry*, **143**, 323–326.

Ekdawi, M. Y. and Conning, A. M. (1994) *Psychiatric Rehabilitation: A Practical Guide*. Chapman & Hall, London.

Ellis, R. and Whittington, D. (1981) *A Guide to Social Skill Training*. Croom Helm, London.

Erikson, E. (1977) *Childhood and Society*. Triad Paladin, St Albans.

Fairgrieve, E. (1996) The impact of sensory integration therapy in the United Kingdom and Ireland: a developmental perspective. *British Journal of Occupational Therapy*, **59**, 452–456.

Fidler, G. S. and Fidler, J. W. (1963) *Occupational therapy: a communication process in psychiatry*. Macmillan, New York.

Fidler, G. and Fidler, J. (1983) Doing and becoming: the occupational therapy experience. In G. Kielhofner (ed.), *Health through occupation: theory and practice in occupational therapy*. F. A. Davis Company, Philadelphia, PA.

Finlay, L. (1993) *Groupwork*. Chapman & Hall, London.

Finlay, L. (1996) Groupwork. In J. Creek (ed.), *Occupational Therapy and Mental Health*, 2nd edn. Churchill Livingstone, Edinburgh.

Finlay, L. (1997) Evaluating research articles. *British Journal of Occupational Therapy*, **60**, 205–208.

Fisher, A., Murray, E. and Bundy, A. (1991) *Sensory Integration: Theory and Practice.* Davis, Philadelphia, PA.

Fisher, A. G. (1994) *Assessment Of Motor And Process Skills (Version 8.0) – Unpublished Test Manual.* Colorado State University, Fort Collins, CO.

Fleming, M. H. (1991) The therapist with the three-track mind. *American Journal of Occupational Therapy*, **45**, 1007–1014.

Forsyth, K. (1995) *A User's Guide to the Assessment of Communication and Interaction Skills.* The University of Illinois, Chicago, IL.

Fossey, E. (1996) Using the Occupational Performance History Interview (OPHI): therapists' reflections. *British Journal of Occupational Therapy*, **59**, 223–228.

Foto, M. (1996) Outcome studies: the what, why, how and when. *American Journal of Occupational Therapy*, **5**, 87–88.

Gibson, S. A. (1996) Horticulture as a therapeutic medium. *British Journal of Therapy and Rehabilitation*, **3**, 203–209.

Hagedorn, R. (1992) *Occupational Therapy: Foundations for Practice.* Churchill Livingstone, Edinburgh.

Hagedorn, R. (1996) *Occupational Therapy: Perspectives and Processes.* Churchill Livingstone, Edinburgh.

Hammond, A. (1996) Functional and health assessments used in rheumatology occupational therapy: a review and United Kingdom survey. *British Journal of Occupational Therapy*, **59**, 254–259.

Hansen, R. A. and Atchinson, B. (eds), (1993) Conditions in occupational therapy: effects on occupational performace. Williams and Wilkins, Baltimore, MD.

Harries, P. and Caan, A. W. (1994) What do psychiatric inpatients and ward staff think about occupational therapy? *British Journal of Occupational Therapy*, **57**, 219–233.

Helfrich, C., Kielhofner, G. and Mattingley, C. (1994) Volition as narrative: an understanding of motivation in chronic illness. *American Journal of Occupational Therapy*, **42**, 311–317.

Hemphill, B. J. (ed.) (1982) *The Evaluation Process in Psychiatric Occupational Therapy.* Slack, Thorofare, NJ.

Holden, U. and Woods, R. T. (1988) *Reality Orientation*, 2nd edn. Churchill Livingstone, Edinburgh.

Hopkins, H. (1983) An historical perspective on occupational therapy. In H. L. Hopkins and H. D. Smith (eds), *Willard and Spackman's Occupational Therapy*, 6th edn. Lippincott, Philadelphia, PA.

Hopkins, H. L. and Tiffany, E. G. (1983) Occupational therapy: a problem-solving process. In H. L. Hopkins and H. D. Smith (eds), *Willard and Spackman's Occupational Therapy*, 6th edn. Lippincott, Philadelphia, PA.

Howell, C. (1986) A controlled trial of goal setting for long-term community psychiatric patients, *British Journal of Occupational Therapy*, **49**, 264–268.

Hutchings, S., Comins, J. and Offiler, J. (1991) *The Social Skills Handbook.* Winslow Press, Oxford.

Jeffrey, L. (1995) Play therapy. In J. Creek (ed.), *Occupational Therapy and Mental Health*, 2nd edn. Churchill Livingstone, Edinburgh.

Jenkins, M. and Brotherton, C. (1995) In search of a theoretical framework for practice, part 1. *British Journal of Occupational Therapy*, **58**, 280–285.

Jenkins, M., Mallett, J., O'Neill, C., McFadden, M. and Baird, H. (1995) Insights into 'practice' communication: an interactional approach. *British Journal of Occupational Therapy*, **57**, 297–302.

Jennings, S. (ed.) (1987) *Dramatherapy: Theory and Practice for Teachers and Clinicians*. Croom Helm, London.

Kaplan, K. (1986) The directive group: short term treatment for psychiatric patients with a minimal level of functioning. *American Journal of Occupational Therapy*, **40**, 474–481.

Kaplan, K. and Kielhofner, G. (1989) *Occupational Case Analysis Interview and Rating Scale*. Slack, Thorofare, NJ.

Kaur, D., Seager, M. and Orrell, M. (1996) Occupation or therapy? The attitudes of mental health professionals. *British Journal of Occupational Therapy*, **59**, 319–322.

Keable, D. (1996) Managing stress. In M. Willson (ed.), *Occupational Therapy in Short-Term Psychiatry*. Churchill Livingstone, Edinburgh.

Kielhofner, G. (1982) Qualitative research: part one paradigmatic grounds and issues of reliability and validity. *The Occupational Therapy Journal of Research*, **2**, 67–79.

Kielhofner, G. (ed.) (1983) *Health through Occupation – Theory and Practice in Occupational Therapy*. F. A. Davis, Philadelphia, PA.

Kielhofner, G. (ed.) (1985) *A Model of Human Occupation – Theory And Application*. Williams & Wilkins, Baltimore, MD.

Kielhofner, G. (1992) *Conceptual Foundations of Occupational Therapy*. F. A. Davis, Philadelphia, PA.

Kielhofner, G. (ed.) (1995) *Human Occupation: Theory and Application*, 2nd edn. Williams & Wilkins, Baltimore, MD.

Kielhofner, G. and Neville, A. (1983) *The Modified Interest Checklist*. Unpublished manuscript. University of Illinois, Chicago, IL.

Kielhofner, G., Henry, A. and Walens, D. (1989) *A User's Guide to the Occupational History Interview*. American Occupational Therapy Association, Rockville, MD.

Kinebanian, A. and Stomph, M. (1992) Cross cultural occupational therapy: a critical reflection. *American Journal of Occupational Therapy*, **46**, 751–757.

Klyczek, J. and Mann, W. (1986) Therapeutic modality comparisons in day treatment. *American Journal of Occupational Therapy*, **40**, 606–611.

Kortman, B. (1994) The eye of the beholder: models in occupational therapy. *Australian Occupational Therapy Journal*, **41**, 115–122.

Kremer, E. R. H., Nelson, D. and Duncombe, L. (1984) Effects of selected activities on affective meaning in psychiatric patients. *American Journal of Occupational Therapy*, **38**, 552–528.

Lacey, J. H. (1984) Time-limited individual and group treatment for bulimia. In D. Garner and P. Garfinkel (eds), *Handbook of Psychotherapy for Anorexia and Bulimia*. Guildford Press, New York.

Laver, A. J. and Hutchinson, S. (1994) The performance and experience of normal elderly people on the COTNAB. *British Journal of Occupational Therapy*, **57**, 137–142.

Law, M., Baptiste, S. and Mills, (1995) Client-centred practice: what does it mean and does it make a difference? *Canadian Journal of Occupational Therapy*, **62**, 250–257.

Law, M., Baptiste, S., Carswell-Opzoomer, A., McColl, M. A., Polatajko, H. and Pollock, N. (1991) *Canadian Occupational Performance Measure*. Canadian Association of Occupational Therapists Publications, Toronto.

Law, M., Baptiste, S., Carswell-Opzoomer, A., McColl, M. A., Polatajko, H. and Pollock, N. (1994) *Canadian Occupational Performance Measure*, 2nd edn. Canadian Association of Occupational Therapists Publication, Toronto.

Levine, R. E. and Gitlin, L. N. (1993) A model to promote activity competence in elders. *American Journal of Occupational Therapy*, **47**, 147–153.

Maslow, A. H. (1954) *Motivation and Personality*. Harper & Row, New York.

Matsutsuyu, J. (1969) The interest checklist. *American Journal of Occupational Therapy*, **23**, 323–328.

Mattingly, C. (1991) The narrative nature of clinical reasoning. *American Journal of Occupational Therapy*, **45**, 998–1005.

Mattingly, C. and Fleming, M. H. (1994) *Clinical Reasoning: Forms of Enquiry in a Therapeutic Practice*. Davis, Philadelphia, PA.

Mayers, C. (1990) A philosophy unique to occupational therapy. *British Journal of Occupational Therapy*, **53**, 379–380.

McAvoy, E. (1991) The use of ADL indices by occupational therapists. *British Journal of Occupational Therapy*, **54**, 383–385.

McDermott, A. (1988) The effect of three group formats on group interaction patterns. In D. Gibson (ed.), *Group Process and Structure in Psycho-Social Occupational Therapy*. Haworth Press, New York.

Mead, M. (1934) *Mind, Self and Society*. University of Chicago Press, Chicago, IL.

Mitchell, L. (1977) *Simple Relaxation*. John Murray, London.

Mocellin, G. (1995) Occupational therapy: a critical overview, part 1. *British Journal of Occupational Therapy*, **58**, 502–506.

Mocellin, G. (1996) Occupational therapy: a critical overview, part 2. *British Journal of Occupational Therapy*, **59**, 11–16.

Moore, C. and Bracegirdle, H. (1994) The effects of a short-term low-intensity exercise programme on the psychological wellbeing of community-dwelling elderly women. *British Journal of Occupational Therapy*, **57**, 213–216.

Moreno, J. L. (1953) *Who Shall Survive?*, revised edn. Beacon House, New York.

Mosey, A. C. (1973) *Activities Therapy*. Raven Press, New York.

Mosey, A. C. (1985) Eleanor Clarke Slagle Lecture: a monistic or pluralistic approach to professional identity? *American Journal of Occupational Therapy*, **39**, 504–509.

Mosey, A. C. (1974) An alternative: the biopsychosocial model. *American Journal of Occupational Therapy*, **28**, 137–140.

Mosey, A. C. (1981) *Occupational Therapy: Configuration of a Profession*. Raven Press, New York.

Mosey, A. C. (1970) *Three Frames of Reference for Mental Health*. Slack, Thorofare, NJ.

Mosey, A. C. (1986) *Psychosocial Components of Occupational Therapy*. Raven Press, New York.

Munroe, H. (1995) Perspectives on clinical reasoning. *British Journal of Therapy and Rehabilitation*, **2**, 313–317.

Nichol, M. (1984) Constructive activities. In M. Willson (ed.), *Occupational Therapy in Short-term Psychiatry*. Churchill Livingstone, Edinburgh.

Nihara, K., Leland, H. and Lambert, N. (1993) *Adaptive Behaviour Scale – Residential and Community*, 2nd edn. American Association on Mental Retardation, Austin, TX.

Oakley, F. (1981) *The Role Checklist*. National Institutes of Health, Bethesda, MD.

Oakley, F., Kielhofner, G., Barris, R. and Reichler, R. K. (1986) The Role Checklist: development and empirical assessment of reliability. *Occupational Therapy Journal of Research*, **6**, 157–170.

Oxley, C. (1995) Work and work programmes for clients with mental health problems,

British Journal of Occupational Therapy, **58**, 465–468.

Pattie, A. H. and Gilleard, C. J. (1979) *Clifton Assessment Procedures for the Elderly (CAPE)*. Hodder & Stoughton, London.

Perri, M. G. (1985) Self-change strategies for the control of smoking, obesity and problem drinking. In Shiffman, S. and Wills, T. A. (eds), *Coping and Substance Abuse*, Academic Press, Orlando, FL.

Platts, L. (1993) Social role valorisation and the model of human occupation: a comparative analysis for work with people with learning disability in the community. *British Journal of Occupational Therapy*, **56**, 278–282.

Polimeni-Walker, I., Wilson, K. and Jewens, R. (1992) Reasons for participating in occupational therapy groups: perceptions of adult psychiatric in-patients and occupational therapists. *Canadian Journal of Occupational Therapy*, **59**, 240–247.

Predretti, L. W. (1996) Occupational performance: a model for practice in physical dysfunction. In L. W. Predretti (ed.), *Occupational Therapy: Practice Skills for Physical Dysfunction*, 4th edn. Mosby, St Louis, MO.

Primeau, L. (1996) Work and leisure: transcending the dichotomy. *American Journal of Occupational Therapy*, **50**, 569–577.

Ravetz, C. (1984) Leisure. In M. Willson (ed.), *Occupational Therapy in Short-Term Psychiatry*. Churchill Livingstone, Edinburgh.

Reed, K. (1984) *Models Of Practice In Occupational Therapy*. Williams & Wilkins, Baltimore, MD.

Reed, K. L. and Sanderson, S. R. (1983) *Concepts Of Occupational Therapy*, 2nd edn. Williams & Wilkins, Baltimore, MD.

Reilly, M. (ed.) (1974) *Play as Exploratory Learning*. Sage, Beverly Hills, CA.

Reilly, M. (1962) Occupational therapy can be one of the greatest ideas of 20th century medicine, *American Journal of Occupational Therapy*, **16**, 1–9.

Richards, S. (1996) Personal communication.

Robinson, S. E. and Fisher, A. G. (1996) A study to examine the relationship of the Assessment of Motor and Process Skills (AMPS) to other tests of cognition and function. *British Journal of Occupational Therapy*, **59**, 260–263.

Rogers, J. C. (1983) Eleanor Clarke Slagle Lecture: clinical reasoning: the ethics, science, and art, *American Journal of Occupational Therapy*, **37**, 601–606.

Rogers, C. (1961) *On Becoming a Person*. Houghton Mifflin, Boston, MA.

Rogers, C. (1970) *Client-centered Therapy*. Constable, London.

Rutter, R. (1995) Clinical implications of attachment concepts: retrospect and prospect. *Journal of Child Psychology and Psychiatry*, **36**, 549–571.

Ryan, S. (1995) The study and application of clinical reasoning research. *British Journal of Therapy and Rehabilitation*, **2**, 265–271.

Schell, B. A. and Cervero, R. M. (1993) Clinical reasoning in occupational therapy: an integrative review. *American Journal of Occupational Therapy*, **47**, 605–610.

Schon, D. (1983) *The Reflective Practitioner: How Professionals Think in Action*. Basic Books, New York.

Sloan, R. L., Downie, C., Hornby, J. and Pentland, B. (1991) Routine screening of brain damaged patients: a comparison of the Rivermead Perceptual Assessment Battery and the Chessington Occupational Therapy Neurological Battery. *Clinical Rehabilitation*, **5**, 265–272.

Smith, L. A. (1996) How do other professions view occupational therapy? *British Journal of Occupational Therapy*, **49**, 51–52.

Smith, N., Kielhofner, G. and Watts, J. (1986) The relationship between volition, activity pattern and life satisfaction in the elderly. *American Journal of Occupational Therapy*, **40**, 278–283.

Spreadbury, P. and Cook, S. (1996) Quality assurance and clinical audit. In J. Creek (ed.), *Occupational Therapy and Mental Health*, 2nd edn. Churchill Livingstone, Edinburgh.

Stevens, R. (1991) Personal identity. In *Identities and Interaction – Society and Social Science: A Foundation Course*. The Open University, Milton Keynes.

Stewart, A. (1990) Research. In J. Creek (ed.), *Occupational Therapy and Mental Health*, 2nd edn. Churchill Livingstone, Edinburgh.

Stockwell, R., Powell, A., Bhat, A. and Evans, C. (1987) Patients' views of occupational therapy in a therapeutic milieu. *British Journal of Occupational Therapy*, **50**, 406–410.

Toates, F. (1996) The embodied self: a biological perspective. In R. Stevens (ed.), *Understanding the Self*. The Open University and Sage, London.

Toomey, M., Nicholson, D. and Carswell, A. (1995) The clinical utility of the Canadian Occupational Performance Measure. *Canadian Journal of Occupational Therapy*, **62**, 242–249.

Velozo, C., Kielhofner, B. and Fisher, G. (1992) *A User's guide to the Worker Role Interview*. The University of Illinois at Chicago, Chicago, IL.

Waller, D. (1993) *Group interactive art therapy: its use in training and treatment*. Routledge, London.

Warr, P. (1987) Work, *Unemployment and Mental Health*. Clarendon Press, Oxford.

Waters, D. (1995) Recovering from a depressive episode using the Canadian Occupational Performance Measure. *Canadian Journal of Occupational Therapy*, **62**, 278–282.

Whiting, S., Lincoln, N. B., Bhavnani, G. and Cockburn, J. (1985) *The Rivermead Perceptual Assessment Battery*. NFER-Nelson, Windsor.

Wilkinson, S. (1988) The role of reflexivity in feminist psychology. *Women's Studies International Forum*, 11, 493–502.

Wolfensberger, W. (1993) *The Principle of Normalisation in Human Sciences*, 2nd edn. National Institute on Mental Retardation, Toronto.

Yerxa, E. J. (1967) Eleanor Clarke Slagle Lecture: authentic occupational therapy. *American Journal of Occupational Therapy*, **21**, 1–9.

Yerxa, E. J. (1979) *The Philosophical Base of Occupational Therapy in 2001 AD*. American Occupational Therapy Association, Rockville, MD.

Yerxa, E. J. (1983a) The occupational therapist as a researcher. In Hopkins, H. L. and Smith, H. D. (eds), *Willard and Spackman's Occupational Therapy*, 6th edn. Lippincott, Philadelphia, PA.

Yerxa, E. J. (1983b) Audacious values: the energy source for occupational therapy practice. In Kielhofner, G. (ed.), *Health through Occupation – Theory and Practice in Occupational Therapy*. Davis, Philadelphia, PA.

Yerxa, E. J. (1986) *In Target 2000; Promoting Excellence in Education*. American Occupational Therapy Association, Rockville, MD.

Yerxa, E. J. (1987) Quotations taken from talks given by Professor E. Yerxa at a conference in Exeter on *Occupational Therapy: A Foundation for Practice*, 2–4 April.

Young, M. and Quinn, E. (1992) *Theories and Principles of Occupational Therapy*. Churchill Livingstone, Edinburgh.

Zimbardo, P. G. (1990) Pathology of imprisonment. In J. Anderson and M. Ricci (eds) *Society and Social Science: A Reader*. The Open University, Milton Keynes.

Index